100 Questions & Answers About High Blood Pressure (Hypertension)

Raymond R. Townsend, MD

Professor of Medicine
University of Pennsylvania
Philadelphia, PA

JONES AND BARTLETT PUBLISHERS
Sudbury, Massachusetts
BOSTON   TORONTO   LONDON   SINGAPORE

World Headquarters
Jones and Bartlett Publishers
40 Tall Pine Drive
Sudbury, MA 01776
978-443-5000
info@jbpub.com
www.jbpub.com

Jones and Bartlett Publishers
Canada
6339 Ormindale Way
Mississauga, Ontario L5V 1J2
CANADA

Jones and Bartlett Publishers
International
Barb House, Barb Mews
London W6 7PA
UK

Jones and Bartlett's books and products are available through most bookstores and online booksellers. To contact Jones and Bartlett Publishers directly, call 800-832-0034, fax 978-443-8000, or visit our website, www.jbpub.com.

Substantial discounts on bulk quantities of Jones and Bartlett's publications are available to corporations, professional associations, and other qualified organizations. For details and specific discount information, contact the special sales department at Jones and Bartlett via the above contact information or send an email to specialsales@jbpub.com.

Copyright © 2008 by Jones and Bartlett Publishers, Inc.

ISBN 13: 978-0-7637-5351-1
ISBN 10: 0-7637-5351-3

Cover images: © Shutterstock

The authors, editor, and publisher have made every effort to provide accurate information. However, they are not responsible for errors, omissions, or for any outcomes related to the use of the contents of this book and take no responsibility for the use of the products and procedures described. Treatments and side effects described in this book may not be applicable to all people; likewise, some people may require a dose or experience a side effect that is not described herein. Drugs and medical devices are discussed that may have limited availability controlled by the Food and Drug Administration (FDA) for use only in a research study or clinical trial. Research, clinical practice, and government regulations often change the accepted standard in this field. When consideration is being given to use of any drug in the clinical setting, the health care provider or reader is responsible for determining FDA status of the drug, reading the package insert, and reviewing prescribing information for the most up-to-date recommendations on dose, precautions, and contraindications, and determining the appropriate usage for the product. This is especially important in the case of

CIP Data was not available at time of printing.

Production Credits
Executive Publisher: Christopher Davis
Acquisitions Editor: Janice Hackenberg
Production Director: Amy Rose
Associate Production Editor: Rachel Rossi
Associate Editor: Kathy Richardson

Associate Marketing Manager: Rebecca Wasley
Manufacturing Buyer: Therese Connell
Composition: Appingo Publishing Services
Cover Design: Jon Ayotte
Printing and Binding: Malloy, Inc.
Cover Printing: Malloy, Inc.

6048

Printed in the United States of America
11 10 09 08 07   10 9 8 7 6 5 4 3 2 1

I would like to dedicate this work to my mentors Don DiPette (currently Dean of the University of South Carolina School of Medicine), Alfred Sellers (Cardiology Faculty at my current institution—the University of Pennsylvania) and Karl Engelman (Retired Penn faculty member now engaged in volunteer medical services in South Carolina) who help guide me at critical points in my career. To the nurse practitioners Liz Weber, Terri Paschetag, Linda Palmquist and Jinny Ford who added so much to patient care through their labors with me. What a privilege it has been to work with these gals. To the patients who have taught me so much about high blood pressure through sharing their experiences with me over these many years. And to my wife of 29 years, Arlene, who deserves sainthood as a reward for the many times I came home a little later than other husbands. She has been an anchor in the rough times of these journeys.

CONTENTS

Preface   **vii**

Part I: The Basics   **1**

Questions 1–22 provide background information regarding blood pressure and hypertension, including:

- What is hypertension?
- What causes hypertension?
- What happens to my blood pressure when I am sleeping?

Part II: Lifestyle/Exercise   **37**

Questions 23–41 explore a number of inquiries about day-to-day life with high blood pressure, such as:

- What kinds of lifestyle changes do I need to make if I have hypertension?
- How does stress affect my blood pressure, and by how much?
- Does acupuncture lower blood pressure?

Part III: Dietary   **61**

Questions 42–46 cover special dietary concerns you may have regarding your blood pressure, such as:

- Does alcohol lower blood pressure?
- My neighbor takes fish oil capsules to reduce her blood pressure. Do they work?
- I was told not to eat grapefruit or drink grapefruit juice because of the type of blood pressure medicine I take. Why is that?

Part IV: Medication-Related   **67**

Questions 47–75 discuss matters surrounding medical treatments available to patients with hypertension, including:

- How will I know when I need to start taking blood pressure medication, especially if my blood pressure fluctuates?
- I don't like swallowing pills. What can I do to get my medicine down?
- How does a doctor decide which medication to give to someone with high blood pressure?

Part V: Doctor/Provider Issues 105

Questions 76–86 are concerned with issues between you and your doctor/ provider, such as:
- What do I do when different doctors tell me to take different medications?
- How can I have confidence that my doctor will listen to me if I have side effects?
- My upper arm is relatively large, so my doctor takes my blood pressure near my wrist. Is that accurate?

Part VI: High Blood Pressure & Other Health Problems/Issues 121

Questions 87–99 explore a variety of other health concerns that are linked to your hypertension, including:
- Why do blood pressure readings have to be even lower than the readings for other people with hypertension when I have diabetes?
- I have bad allergies. What can I take for them that will not interfere with my blood pressure?
- How does high blood pressure affect the kidneys?
- I am nursing my new baby now. What medications can I take for my blood pressure while nursing?

Appendix   **141**

Glossary   **149**

Index   **157**

High blood pressure is common. Books on it are pretty common too. Why publish another book on it, and why read this one in particular? Two reasons.

One: No one has the market cornered on this; there is always more to learn. Two: This book is not just a series of 100 factoids about hypertension. Woven into this work are 20+ years of experience, failure, success, practicality and just a sprinkle of humor which may provide a little encouragement for people who have high blood pressure, or are related to someone who has it.

Ray Townsend
August 2007

PART ONE

The Basics

What is blood pressure, and why is it important?

Why are there two numbers in a
blood pressure reading?

What is hypertension?

More . . .

1. What is blood pressure, and why is it important?

The amount of pressure generated by the heart with each heartbeat has to satisfy the needs of the body and not overwork the heart in the process. That's where the delicate balancing act comes into play.

Blood pressure, like any pressure, is a measure of force. In this case, the force is the power directing blood to flow through the body's circulation. We need a certain amount of force so that the blood can deliver oxygen and other nutrients to our tissues and take away the waste products. Simply put, without blood pressure there would be no delivery of fuel or other essential items to our heart, brain, kidneys, and other organs. The reason blood pressure is so important is related to where it comes from—that is, the heart.

The heart is the sole generator of the force governing the blood pressure. That's a big job, and one with no mandatory two-week vacation for each one year's worth of service! Moreover, the heart has to deliver blood to itself, a challenging feat when it's busy contracting and sending blood elsewhere. That task requires a delicate balance of work, relax, refuel; then work, relax, refuel; and repeat over, and over, and over. Multiply this cycle by 70 beats per minute, 60 minutes per hour, 24 hours per day, 365 days per year, and perhaps 80 years if you're lucky, and it works out to nearly 300 million heartbeats per human life. And that rate does not allow for exercise and other activities that increase your heart rate. Thus the trick is for the heart is to deliver needed nutrients to the body, and to itself, in sickness and in health, at exercise and at rest, whether eating or fasting, and—well, you get the idea.

The amount of pressure generated by the heart with each heartbeat has to satisfy the needs of the body and not overwork the heart in the process. That's where the delicate balancing act comes into play. When pressure is either too low or too high, trouble begins. The rest of the questions in this book address these issues in greater detail.

2. Why are there two numbers in a blood pressure reading?

The two numbers in a blood pressure reading correspond to the highest and lowest pressures generated by (1) the heart and (2) the circulation with each heartbeat. Because the heart needs a break in between each heartbeat, it isn't possible to generate a continuous pressure.

The upper number in the blood pressure reading indicates the amount of force the heart uses to "push" blood into the big arteries, such as the aorta. These big arteries store this blood for a moment and then dole it out to the rest of the body, as continuously and smoothly as possible. In this way, the big arteries function like a cushion for each heartbeat, converting the pulsations of each heartbeat into a continuous flow of nourishment to the tissues.

The lower number in the blood pressure reading represents the amount of **resistance** to the flow of the blood. This lower pressure number reflects how the body determines where blood should go at any particular time. To see how this works, consider this analogy: Suppose you are working in the central waterworks of a busy city. You have a bunch of separate districts that need water, but different amounts and at different times. Perhaps the carwash district needs lots of water between 8 and 9 A.M. when people are going to work and running their vehicles through the carwash, with another peak occurring at 4 to 5 P.M. as they are returning home. The peak water needs for the restaurant district occur at 11 A.M. to 1 P.M. (lunch) and 6 to 10 P.M. (dinner). You can't supply water full force to all areas at the same time, so you ration it out by adjusting the volume of water you send to any one area through a faucet or spigot system.

This is what the lower number in the blood pressure reading represents: It indicates what happens when all of the body's "spigots" are turned on or off at any one time. When you exercise, for

Resistance

A term carried over from the world of physics. In electricity there are three forces. There is a certain amount of moving force, a certain amount of flow, and certain amount of resistance to flow that are related by this formula: Force = Flow * Resistance. (The * is a math symbol for multiplication. Reading this aloud you would say "Force equals flow times resistance"). See Vascular Resistance.

Hypertension

Also called high blood pressure. Hypertension is a circumstance in which a person's blood pressure has been shown to be consistently at or above 140/90 mm Hg. Hypertension is a leading risk factor for stroke, heart disease, kidney disease and peripheral circulation problems.

Actuaries

Tables of life insurance company data that typically evaluate factors involved in risks of dying. These factors include things like cigarette use, blood pressure and cholesterol levels.

mm Hg

Abbreviation for millimeters (mm) of mercury (chemical symbol is Hg), the units in which blood pressure is measured.

example, your muscles need more blood to handle the increased need for oxygen and nutrients (and waste product production). The lower blood pressure number typically falls during exercise as you "open the spigots" to the muscle tissues; the spigots close down again about 20 minutes after you have turned off your favorite Aerobics Diva and headed for the showers.

Both numbers in the blood pressure reading are important, and both are used in making the diagnosis of hypertension as well as adjusting therapy in people with hypertension.

3. What is hypertension?

The definition of **hypertension** is a somewhat arbitrary one. Once it became possible to measure blood pressure accurately (around the beginning of the twentieth century), the group with the greatest interest in the risk associated with high blood pressure was actually the life insurance industry. Consequently, **actuaries** determined what level of blood pressure was considered "hypertension." They made this determination through a logical sequence of measuring blood pressures in literally hundreds of thousands of people. These studies indicated that the risk of death did not suddenly begin at any particular level of blood pressure, but that people with blood pressure levels such as 140/90 mm Hg had a substantially higher risk of death than people with values such as 115/70 mm Hg. Bear in mind that this issue was settled long before any blood pressure medication was available. By the middle of the twentieth century, life insurance data (including mortality statistics) were available on more than 250,000 people. Perhaps one of the most sobering statistics is that if you were a 40-year-old man who was diagnosed with hypertension in 1940, depending on the level of blood pressure you had at the time of diagnosis, your lifespan could be as short as a year or as long as 15 or perhaps 20 years.

Today a diagnosis of hypertension still uses the same threshold values established by the insurance industry: 140/90 mm Hg (**mm Hg** is the unit used for blood pressure; "mm" is an abbreviation for "millimeters," and "Hg" is the chemical symbol for mercury, the stuff that was used in the little glass tube that actually measures the blood pressure). It is important to understand that hypertension is a disorder of pressure in the blood vessels, not an issue with being tense or distressed easily. Thus, when we say that someone is "hyper," we are referring to a stereotype characterized by nervousness and jitters. We are *not* talking about the person's blood pressure!

Blood pressure tends to be somewhat variable, so doctors generally make the diagnosis of high blood pressure only after they have checked it on several different occasions. The exception to this rule is when someone presents with very high levels of blood pressure—for example, 180/120 mm Hg. In that case, the physician will usually initiate therapy promptly.

Oddly enough, the diagnosis of hypertension can be a blessing in disguise. Because hypertension is often without symptoms, it has earned the name of "silent killer." Being aware of having hypertension is the first step in managing it. If you have hypertension, you're in good company: Millions of people have hypertension. Fortunately, thanks to the many effective treatments now available for this disease, the gloomy statistics quoted earlier are no longer the norm. The abundance of information we have on lifestyle and medication therapies can usually be tailored successfully to manage your blood pressure, often with minimal bother. So cheer up, and read on!

Hypertension is a disorder of pressure in the blood vessels, not an issue with being tense or distressed easily.

The Basics

4. How many readings of my blood pressure are necessary before I can be sure I have been correctly diagnosed as having high blood pressure?

In my practice, I sometimes tell my patients that managing hypertension is like trying to grasp an invisible python coated with Vaseline. Blood pressure levels vary quite a bit, as anyone who has taken a bunch of them at home will tell you. Just when you think you've got everything under control, a stray high or low value creeps in. The lesson we have learned from this management challenge is to perform multiple readings. In fact, the gurus who tell us how to diagnose hypertension insist that we take several blood pressure measurements at any one visit, and that we do so on at least three occasions. We diagnose hypertension when the average of all these readings is more than 140/90 mm Hg.

"But what if my average blood pressure is 139/89 mm Hg?", you might ask. Not to worry—doctors who treat hypertension have a category for everything! We consider values of the upper number in the blood pressure reading between 120 and 139 mm Hg (inclusive) to be **pre-hypertension.** Most people with values in that range will eventually slip over the threshold of 140/90 mm Hg and develop hypertension in the next few years. However, some highly motivated folk may make significant lifestyle adjustments (covered in later questions) in an attempt to stave off this outcome.

Pre-hypertension

A term used when someone's blood pressure is consistently 120-139 mm Hg in the upper number (see Systolic) and/or 80-89 mm Hg in the lower number (see Diastolic).

In some special situations, hypertension may be diagnosed based on a single blood pressure visit. This diagnosis is usually made because the level of blood pressure is considerably high, and in such cases it may not be wise to wait a couple of weeks to take repeat readings before beginning therapy. Question 3 cited a blood pressure reading of 180/120 mm Hg as an example, but in some cases lower values (even on a single visit) would be considered hypertension.

The threshold values of 140/90 mmHg used to diagnose hypertension apply to adults, specifically people 18 years of age or older. Different values are used for children. In children, hypertension is diagnosed based on height- and gender-specific guidelines (more on this issue in Question 5). The appendix in this book titled "Literature and Other Sources of Information" identifies a Web site that provides the tables that are used to make the diagnosis of high normal blood pressure and hypertension in children.

Pop quiz: How much attention have you been paying to Question 4? Let's see! How many sets of blood pressure readings are necessary before a diagnosis of hypertension is made in most people?

(a) It depends on your age.
(b) It depends on your parent's age.
(c) Usually three.
(d) Hold that thought—I'll answer this in a minute (soon as I reread Question 4).

5. What causes hypertension?

Great question, but bad answer. The truth is that we often don't know why a person develops hypertension. We know about a lot of things that *affect* blood pressure levels, but we are still trying to figure what *causes* high blood pressure in most people. What we know so far is this:

- There appears to be a genetic link. (Hypertension is more common in families where hypertension is present in the parents.)
- There appears to be an environmental link. (For example, hypertension is more common when there is free access to salt.)

We know about a lot of things that affect blood pressure levels, but we are still trying to figure what causes high blood pressure in most people.

That said, some things clearly predict the onset of hypertension in certain people. One of the most reliable indicators of who will have hypertension someone is a person's weight. Hypertension occasionally occurs in lean people, but it is more common in people who are overweight, and it will often occur at a younger age in people who are overweight. Not only are total calories eaten important, but the relative amounts of minerals consumed as part of the diet seem to play a role in the development of hypertension as well. A diet rich in potassium (which comes from fruits, for example) is less likely to be associated with hypertension than a diet rich in sodium (which is found in foods that come in bags, boxes, and cans).

Lastly, age tends to be a very potent predictor. The prevalence of hypertension in college-age people is probably in the range of 2% to 3%, whereas the prevalence of hypertension in elderly people is in the range of 65% or more.

Currently, scientists believe that hypertension results from a combination of the inherited tendencies we have toward hypertension and the things we eat or don't do (such as exercise regularly). This so-called nature/nurture connection probably applies to many chronic disorders, including hypertension. As you can see, it's a convenient solution: We can blame both our parents and ourselves.

6. How can it be that my blood pressure was always low in the past and now it's high?

If I only had a nickel, for every patient who asked me this question! This is one of the most difficult questions healthcare providers must answer when treating patients with a new onset of hypertension. It's always comforting to receive a pat on the back from the healthcare provider who is impressed with your "low" level of blood pressure. It often comes as a huge surprise when instead of a smile, the healthcare provider shows a frown or look of consternation, followed by the comment, "Did you know your blood pressure is high?" How is such a change possible?

In some people, hypertension is "wired" into their systems much like the timer on an alarm clock. For reasons we wish we understood better, in some people the alarm goes off and their blood pressure—which had been wonderful up to that point—becomes elevated. As mentioned in Question 4, a single high reading may be a fluke. All too commonly, however, it is just the first of several elevated readings in someone who previously had remarkably normal or low levels of blood pressure. Sometimes, there may be a logical explanation for this phenomenon, such as use of certain medications (discussed in later questions). Sometimes, it is associated with substantial weight gain. And sometimes, visiting the "all you can eat" Chinese food buffet and consuming liberal dollops of soy sauce might have been the key.

Physicians will often look for triggers that might have led to a sudden change in blood pressure level, but not uncommonly they come up empty-handed. In other circumstances, a cause may be found weeks or even months after the change in blood pressure occurs, but these cases tend to be the exception rather than the rule. Particularly when a person has a family history of hypertension, it is likely that a sudden change in blood pressure levels, when verified on a few rechecks, will be permanent.

Virginia comments:

My doctors worried when I was in my twenties that my blood pressure was too low. They were always asking me if I felt light-headed or dizzy (I didn't), but when I reached my mid-forties, I was astonished to be diagnosed with hypertension. Now that I am experienced as a nurse practitioner, I frequently see chronic diseases, such as hypertension and diabetes, emerging in this age group. Usually the family history supports these diagnoses.

7. What does high cholesterol have to do with hypertension?

In simple terms, the answer to this question is "guilt by association." One lesson we have learned over the past 50 years is that risk factors for heart disease tend to be partners in crime as well as bedfellows. In other words, if your **cholesterol** level is high, your blood pressure is often high as well, and vice versa. This relationship makes more sense when you think about how common each of these findings is in the general adult population. Blood pressure and cholesterol affect different parts of the blood vessel. Hypertension affects mostly the muscular layer of the blood vessel wall, whereas cholesterol tends to accumulate in the lining of the blood vessel (the innermost part, where the blood is flowing—sometimes sluggishly). When both the cholesterol level and the blood

Cholesterol

A form of lipid important in heart disease. Cholesterol is the basis for sex hormones and bile, but it is also a substance that can accumulate in the lining of blood vessels and cause blockages.

Hormones

Chemicals made by glands like the adrenal glands or the pancreas that signal other tissue to function in a particular manner. For example insulin is a hormone made by the pancreas which, when released into the blood, stimulates the liver (and other tissues) to take up glucose (sugar) from the blood and store it.

Plaque

An area of hardening in the blood vessel.

pressure are elevated, it portends bad news for the circulation if these conditions are left untreated.

In some cases, the buildup of cholesterol in the lining of the blood vessel impairs blood flow to crucial organs such as the kidneys. In this respect, its accumulation can cause or contribute to high blood pressure because the kidneys are uniquely able to release chemicals (**hormones**) that raise blood pressure when their blood flow is reduced—for example, by the presence of cholesterol **plaque** in the main kidney arteries.

Another way that cholesterol levels and blood pressure are related is that diet affects both. A diet that is rich in animal fats and salt (a kind of one–two punch in the blood vessel) contributes to increases in both cholesterol levels and blood pressure. Remember that last rib-eye steak smothered in a savory mushroom gravy? And that third glass of choice Merlot? (Oops, now we're getting ahead of ourselves—that's the subject of Question 23.)

Lastly, the blood cholesterol concentration acts as a kind of "poor man's barometer" for the body's energy balance. When the amount of energy (that is, calories) provided by the diet is more than the amount of energy expended (for example, through exercise), the excess is stored in fat tissues. One of the markers of this imbalance in **lipid** (fat) accumulation is an increase in both cholesterol and **triglyceride** (cholesterol's favorite dance partner; triglycerides are one of the important fats involved in hardening of the arteries) levels. As mentioned before, such an increase in stored calories—in other words, an increase in body weight—also contributes to high blood pressure.

Lipids

Generally considered these are the fats (or triglycerides) and cholesterol found in blood. Higher density lipids are the "good" fats and the lower density lipids are the "bad" fats.

8. What causes blood pressure to change so much during the course of the day?

Consider the job description of your circulatory system. Your blood vessels work together with your heart to deliver nutrients and oxygen to the various tissues of the body; at the same time, the blood also picks up waste products to return to the kidneys, lungs, and liver (among other organs). All in all, the circulation is a remarkable system. If the demand for its services was constant, your blood pressure would not change much throughout the course of the day. However, we eat, sleep, run, and do all sorts of things in the course of an average 24-hour cycle that places many demands on the circulation. As a result, our blood pressure is a dynamic rather than a **static** variable in each of us.

For this reason it's recommended that your blood pressure be checked after you have sat quietly for five minutes. This is necessary for two reasons. First, all of our information on the predictive value of knowing blood pressure, and the results of treating it, is based on blood pressures taken after someone has been sitting quietly for five minutes. Second, sitting quietly allows the system to "settle" to its current value. The effects of day-to-day activity cloud the issue of what blood pressure is doing in terms of the damage it inflicts on someone over the course of his or her lifetime. We know that blood pressure varies based on physical activity, and this variation is a good thing. However, if we want to know how any one person compares to a group of people who have been followed closely to determine the effects of blood pressure on their heart, brain, and kidneys, we must do something to reduce this variability in blood pressure so that we can see clearly what's really "under the hood."

In a recent article in *Parade* magazine, one healthcare expert decried the practice of having patients sit quietly before measuring their blood pressure. He seemed much more interested in what their responses to exercise or other daily activities were. The problem with this approach is that if you run a mile and I run a mile, and then both of us have our blood pressures taken at the finish line, it's extremely unlikely that our blood pressure responses to this exercise will be comparable. If we both sit for five minutes before having our blood pressures measured, however, the blood pressure level obtained can be compared with literally hundreds of

Triglyceride

A type of fat, or lipid, that serves as the principal energy storage form of fat calories in the body. Triglycerides are stored in many tissues, but most notably in fat cells. Triglycerides circulate in the body in a particle called a Very Low Density Lipoprotein or VLDL. When VLDL particles are depleted of their triglycerides, they become Low Density Lipoproteins (LDL) which are very rich in the bad form of cholesterol.

Static

This term refers to something that is steady or unchanging.

The Basics

thousands of other patients' values, and good decisions can then be made—especially when it comes to selecting a blood pressure medication.

One of the biggest challenges when taking care of patients with hypertension is interpreting their home blood pressure readings. We will have more to say about this issue later, but for now just recognize that the "venial sin" of home blood pressure monitoring is failure to abide by the simple five-minute rule. When I look at pages of home blood pressure readings and see an unexpected degree of variability, I can usually guess (correctly, most of the time) that the patient has not been doing his or her homework, and has been checking blood pressures without this period of rest. Did I mention that you should wait five minutes before taking your blood pressure at home or in the office?

You should wait five minutes before taking your blood pressure at home or in the office.

Virginia comments:

I remember when I was younger and working as a public health nurse, my children were 10 and 16 years old and very skilled in producing guilt feelings. The 10-year-old was often home alone for about one hour (he told everyone he was a latch-key kid) before I arrived home in the late afternoon. I was always feeling stressed and guilty, trying to finish my work on time and then driving as fast as I could to arrive home. Once I happened to take my blood pressure around this time, and it was alarmingly elevated. Later after dinner and relaxing, it was normal again. When I began checking my blood pressure more regularly, I learned just how much physical and mental activity could change the blood pressure within minutes, even seconds. That's why Dr T. says that every-one should rest for at least five minutes so that doctors and nurse practitioners are playing on somewhat of a level field when they make treatment decisions.

9. Should I measure my blood pressure at home? If so, how often?

Now that home blood pressure kits are both inexpensive and relatively reliable, the measurement of blood pressure at home has become much more common than when I started doing hypertension care in nearly 1980s. Whether you should take home readings depends on the following issues:

- *Do you have hypertension?* If you don't, you have less of a need for home blood pressure measurements. However, if you have normal blood pressure but a positive family history of hypertension, than a home blood pressure kit may be an excellent investment.
- *Are you having trouble getting your blood pressure under control?* One of the tug-of-war issues that healthcare providers face when managing hypertensive patients is the classic dilemma of what to do when patients take blood pressure medication but still have uncontrolled levels of blood pressure when measured in the health-care provider's office. In this situation, home blood pressure measurements can be a marvelous addition to office-based care. Of course, they need to be taken correctly to have any value.
- *Are you having any symptoms?* Sometimes patients think that their blood pressure medicines are "hitting" them at times, and are concerned that their blood pressure is "too low." Having the ability to measure blood pressure usually resolves the issue of whether there is a link between blood pressure level and symptoms at the time which the symptoms occur. Naturally, the symptoms never occur in the doctor's office!

How often should you measure blood pressure at home? The answer to this question will depend on a couple of things. If you are in process of having your medications adjusted, then you may need to have blood pressure readings taken two or even four times a day until the dose is settled. I usually prefer

The Basics

to have measurements done in duplicate, and then averaged. Although my patients have great memories, I still ask them to write their measurements down so that I can look at a copybook or some other written record. It's important to note the time of day when blood pressures are taken. Because most of the kits provide a heart rate reading, I like to see that information, too. If someone is fine and his or her blood pressure is well controlled, I typically recommend checking blood pressures every few weeks.

One interesting patient group I've had the privilege to care for has been engineers. These folks take blood pressure monitoring seriously. Often they will bring me not just written records of their blood pressure readings, but also spreadsheets of their values, running averages with standard deviations, and multicolored graphs indicating how they're doing. When I get an e-mail from one of these patients and notice that it has an attachment, I know it's time to refill my coffee cup and sit down for a few minutes! Of course, it's usually not necessary to be quite so thorough. The preferred frequency with which you measure your blood pressure will vary depending on the situation in which the information will be used.

Virginia comments:

Health care in general is changing (i.e., shorter hospitalizations, fewer office visits paid by insurance). More emphasis is placed on teamwork between patient and provider, which inevitably creates more responsibility for the patient to be his or her own advocate. For many reasons, I have found owning a blood pressure kit to be beneficial. It gives me a sense of control over my circumstances. I sometimes get a headache, which is rare for me, but I immediately worry that my blood pressure is "sky-high," even though this is rarely the case. While working as a nurse practitioner in the hypertension program, I have received frantic phone calls from patients who are experiencing nosebleeds and immediately assume that a stroke is right around the corner, when, in fact, the nosebleed is caused by dry air or some other irritation, and the blood pressure is stable. Of course, these blood pressure values must be balanced by taking the blood pressure in the manner that Dr T. has taught you.

Owning and using your blood pressure apparatus routinely will lessen unnecessary phone calls and visits to the doctor, while also providing self-education so that you can differentiate between a normal versus abnormal situation that really does require medical advice or assistance. Your increased knowledge will validate these decisions.

10. What's the best home kit to use to monitor my blood pressure?

This question was a lot easier to answer 15 years ago. Back then, only a handful of kits were available; now there are dozens. Not to worry: *Consumer Reports* has come to the rescue. Every few years this organization does a good job of reviewing home blood pressure kits. You can find the issues of the magazine with these reviews on newsstands, in the library, or online.

There are a few steps you should take before you purchase a kit. First, take a good look at your nondominant arm. In particular, pay attention to the region between your elbow and your shoulder. Herein lies one of the most common pitfalls when choosing a kit to perform home blood pressure measurements. It's the old problem of trying to fit a Cadillac body onto a Volkswagen chassis. Most kits are supplied with a "regular adult"-sized blood pressure cuff. Most adults (well, *many* adults) are overweight, and the regular size (unlike Leggs pantyhose) does not fit all. Consequently, if you're a man who weighs more than 200 pounds or a woman who weighs more than 160 pounds, you should get a kit with a large adult cuff. Sometimes that will mean ordering one from the little coupon tucked inside the box.

Over the years, I have found that the Omron and AND-UA brands of kits do a good job at home blood pressure measurements. (I do not own stock in either company.) These kits include digital cuffs, which are typically self-inflating and self-deflating. In some cases, you attach the cuff, push the button, and voilà—numbers appear as if by magic! In other cases, you attach the cuff and pump it until the machine beeps, indicating that you have put enough air pressure into the system; the machine then takes over from there. Other digital brands are probably just as good, but my experience has been largely with these two.

In general, the upper arm type of kits appear to be the best. Those working at the wrist are decent but not perfect, though they are quite useful in people who have "Popeye-shaped" arms (i.e., funnel-shaped arms, where a typical blood pressure cuff just doesn't cut it). The cuffs that fit on the finger have been largely disappointing. Many reasons underlie their poor performance, but I'll simply say that blood pressure readings taken with the finger cuffs just don't appear as accurate as measurements taken simultaneously with upper arm cuffs.

If you're a do-it-yourself kind of person, you might want to invest in an old-fashioned blood pressure cuff that you inflate yourself and then listen over the artery in your arm with a stethoscope. These manual blood pressure cuffs no longer use mercury, but rather are aneroid models that include a dial-light gauge on the front. They work quite well, but take a bit of practice to get comfortable with their use. Of course, you don't have to worry if the batteries are okay with the manual kits. You do, however, need to make sure the needle on the dial gauge is resting in its little box before using it. **Figure 1** shows an example of a manual blood pressure cuff.

Finally, it's a good idea to have your kit and your technique checked by a healthcare worker once in a while. That way you know you aren't wasting your time when you take readings at home because you'll be assured that ol' Betsy is reading reliably.

The Basics

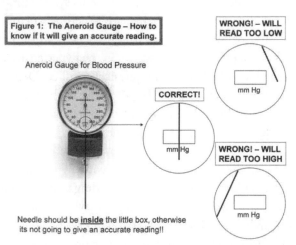

Figure 1   The ANEROID gauge – how to know if it will give an accurate reading

11. My neighbor wore a device that took his blood pressure many times over the course of 24 hours. Do I need to be checked in this way if I have hypertension?

The contraption that takes blood pressure frequently over 24 hours is called an ambulatory blood pressure monitor (ABPM). This device is programmed to take three or four blood pressures every hour while you're awake, and every half hour to one hour while you're asleep. An ABPM is typically used when there is a discrepancy between blood pressures recorded in a doctor's office and those obtained when a patient is at home, at the supermarket, or wherever a blood pressure machine is available. Its principal usage is to diagnose **white coat hypertension.**

White coat hypertension is said to be present when blood pressure readings in the healthcare provider's office are 140/90 mm Hg or higher, but typically 130/85 mm Hg or lower everywhere else. We don't really know why some people react to being in a healthcare setting in this way. It may be related to

White coat hypertension

This term refers to someone whose blood pressure is high in a healthcare setting (like a doctor's office where it has been taken by someone wearing a "white coat") but it is lower at home or when evaluated by ambulatory blood pressure monitoring.

the way in which their involuntary nervous system processes perceived threats to their well-being, such as doctors and nurses. The goal in wearing such a device is to prove that the person's blood pressure levels are not in the hypertensive range when the individual is not the physician's office. Depending on the situation, when the ABPM confirms the presence of white coat hypertension, use of antihypertensive medications may be deferred (at least for the time being).

If you have already been diagnosed with hypertension and perhaps take home blood pressure readings, there would be little reason to wear an ABPM unless you are participating in a research study. For people who are part of such studies, ABPMs do something that just is not practical either in a doctor's office or with home blood pressure kits: They measure your blood pressure while you were sleeping. Most people experience a decrease in their blood pressure when they are sleeping, a phenomenon called dipping. When people fail to show this kind of blood pressure change while asleep, the blood pressure is referred to as non-dipping. Medical research indicates that people who have non-dipping blood pressures tend to have thicker hearts (an undesirable characteristic) and more protein in the urine, both of which can represent target organ effects of hypertension.

Unless the goal is to prove white coat hypertension, most insurers will not cover the costs of ABPM. Nevertheless, wearing an ABPM might be useful in a few other circumstances:

- To demonstrate a relationship between symptoms and blood pressure when it's inconvenient for you to manually check your own blood pressure
- To document extreme variability in blood pressure in some groups of patients (such as those with longstanding diabetes) in whom blood pressure therapy has been challenging

- To look for serious decreases in blood pressure that might not be evident by virtue of symptoms, particularly in older people
- To determine whether blood pressure medications are providing for around-the-clock control and not wearing off too quickly

Fortunately, the 24-hour devices used nowadays are quite light (weighing less than 0.75 pound). When I started using ABPMs in 1984, the recording unit weighed 5 pounds and one of the most common side effects was bruising on the hip from carrying this beast around for 24 hours. Moreover, when the device's alarm went off, everyone in the mall knew someone was wearing an ABPM. The quiet featherweights of today are a vast improvement compared to the noisy mammoths of two decades ago!

12. Does the blood pressure machine in the supermarket give an accurate one-pressure recording?

This is a good question, and I wrote a brief editorial about it a few years ago. Take a good look at the blood pressure equipment before you stick your arm in it. Keep in mind that a device that inflates and deflates at the push of a button can be a significant attraction to young children. On the one hand, it may experience quite a lot of abuse. On the other hand, it may be very well maintained. For these reasons, it's often hard to say whether a blood pressure measurement is accurate.

Perhaps the most useful bit of advice is *caveat emptor* (Latin for "Let the buyer beware"). If possible, have your blood pressure taken twice, with one minute lapsing between the two readings. If the readings are close, within 8 to 10 points (a point is a unit of blood pressure, or 1 mm Hg), the measurement may be accurate. However, few people would stake their medical reputation on managing blood pressure from this kind of device. Also, if you've been walking a lot in the store, then you may simply see the effects of physical activity on your blood pressure, not your real blood pressure (see Question 8). Ideally, you should be able to occupy the device for five minutes without creating a queue of other curious hypertension-information seekers who are waiting patiently for their turn.

The most useful benefit afforded by a store-based system is that if your blood pressure is high, it should prompt you to have it checked again. In my experience, these measurements tend to err on the high side. Rarely do these devices do give someone a false sense of security by reporting low blood pressures in patients whose hypertension is really not controlled. Consequently, we usually interpret values done from stand-alone machines with a grain of salt.

If the supermarket happens to have a pharmacy, some pharmacists are willing to take blood pressures for customers. It doesn't hurt to ask, and the resulting measurement is more likely to be accurate.

13. If my blood pressure is high only when I am at the dentist's office, am I likely to have hypertension?

There's no cure for most people who have high blood pressure, so a diagnosis of hypertension sticks for life. It's worth the effort to be sure that the diagnosis is correct.

You could just as easily replace "dentist's office" with "IRS auditor," "State Trooper pull-over," or a dozen other scenarios in this question. It boils down to a simple issue: "If I am stressed by something, and my blood pressure is elevated during that time, does that mean I have hypertension?" Before reading on, take a look back at Question 9.

The diagnosis of hypertension, common though it is, is important to get right. At the present time, there's no cure for most people who have high blood pressure. Thus, once this condition is identified, the diagnosis sticks for life. Naturally it's worth the effort to be sure—or at least as sure as you can be—that the diagnosis is correct. Multiple readings (and readings taken in a variety of situations, such as in the home and perhaps at the workplace) can really help in this regard.

Why is ensuring that the diagnosis is correct so important? Hypertension is a label, and when people are labeled things begin to happen to them. They may miss a bit more work, and perhaps they feel a little less well. These effects may be subtle, but they have been demonstrated time and again in studies published in the medical literature.

Back to the issue at hand. If your blood pressure is elevated when you are confronted with a situation that scares you (either consciously, such as the way I feel when I see a dentist, or unconsciously, where the terror is felt deep down in the **brain stem** and may not be a conscious or felt emotion), your reaction probably has some medical significance. If your pressure is normal at most other times, then you don't really have hypertension (at least not yet). Nevertheless, half of all people who experience these office-based high blood pressure episodes eventually develop hypertension during the next five years of follow-up. One of the most hotly debated issues in high blood pressure care right now is whether people with these "white coat" or office-based hypertension profiles are at greater risk of target organ effects (such as heart attack and stroke) compared with people whose blood pressure does not behave this way when they are in similar settings. Stay tuned: Maybe the second edition of this book will be able to answer that question!

14. Why is my blood pressure high when I exercise every day, am not overweight, and do not feel stressed?

Blood pressure increases are not restricted to people who eat too much, exercise too little, or do both. Nor are the placid spared. So many processes control blood pressure (because it is such an important facet of the circulation) that there are numerous opportunities for this system to go awry. It's amazing how well

Brain stem

The part of the brain that regulates dilation and constriction of blood vessels.

Servo

A response system connected to other systems and dedicated to serving a purpose, like supporting blood pressure levels. Servos increase their activity when their target system is showing signs of insufficient activity. Servos dial back their influence when the system they serve shows signs of excessive activation.

Adrenal glands

The two small endocrine glands located just above the kidneys. The adrenal glands secrete sex hormones, cortisol, and adrenaline (epinephrine).

Regular exercise and maintaining ideal body weight will go a long way toward protecting the target organs in conjunction with good blood pressure treatment.

the blood pressure system usually works given its complexity, and typically several of the blood pressure **servos** (see **Figure 2,** where each of the four sides is one servo) have to malfunction before blood pressure increases to the point where a diagnosis of hypertension is made. Although being overweight and inactive contributes a great deal to elevated blood pressures, so do a family tendency to develop hypertension, your dietary consumption of minerals (particularly salt), the occasional or perhaps frequent margarita, and many other factors. When asked point-blank, "What makes blood pressure go up?", the truthful healthcare provider will typically respond, "We're not sure." This response applies in at least 90% of all cases. When physicians highlight factors such as obesity and inactivity, we are actually looking at are more associations than direct causes of hypertensions.

Sometimes high blood pressure is actually a symptom of another problem. In that sense, it acts like a blinking arrow directing the physician to look somewhere else. Later questions may reveal where the "somewhere" is, but it is the basic job of healthcare providers to answer three questions when they see a patient with newly diagnosed hypertension:

1. Is the blood pressure increase in this person primary (cause unknown, which accounts for 90% or more of all cases) or secondary (where the cause, when it can be found, is typically the kidney or the **adrenal gland**)?
2. Has the hypertension caused any problems so far?
3. Does the person have cardiovascular risk factors that, in conjunction with hypertension, put him or her at even more risk for having heart disease or stroke in the future?

We'll explore questions 2 and 3 in more detail later in this book.

Don't lose heart in the interim while you are waiting to find a cause for your hypertension. Regular exercise and maintaining ideal body weight will go a long way toward protecting the target organs (brain, heart, and kidney) in conjunction with good blood pressure treatment. Moreover, blood pressure

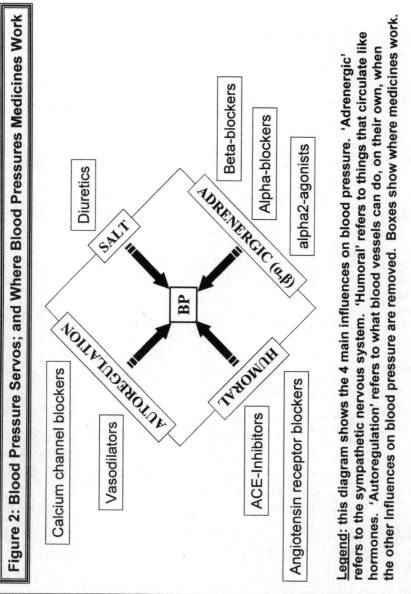

Figure 2: Blood Pressure Servos; and Where Blood Pressures Medicines Work

Legend: this diagram shows the 4 main influences on blood pressure. 'Adrenergic' refers to the sympathetic nervous system. 'Humoral' refers to things that circulate like hormones. 'Autoregulation' refers to what blood vessels can do, on their own, when the other influences on blood pressure are removed. Boxes show where medicines work.

Figure 2   Blood Pressure Servos; and Where Blood Pressure Medicines Work

medications tend to work better in people who are leaner and more active, and it's sometimes possible to use less medication and still achieve and maintain control of blood pressure in such individuals.

15. If my blood pressure was high at the end of my pregnancy but is okay now, do I have hypertension?

Let me cut to the chase and answer the question this way: "You probably do not have hypertension now, but you may develop it in the future."

Many women experience increases in their blood pressure during pregnancy. In particular, four types of hypertension are associated with pregnancy:

Gestational

Having to do with pregnancy.

Preeclampsia

A situation, usually arising after the 20th week of pregnancy, characterized by increased blood pressure, ankle swelling and proteinuria (see Proteinuria) in a pregnant woman.

- Chronic hypertension during pregnancy. Some women have preexisting high blood pressure that persists during pregnancy, though the blood pressure level may fall early on in the pregnancy.
- **Gestational** hypertension. Some women develop blood pressure increases that are transient and last only during the pregnancy (especially the latter part of the pregnancy), only to have their blood pressure level come back to normal after delivery.
- **Preeclampsia.** In some women, blood pressure increases during pregnancy and problems such as swelling in the legs and losing protein in the urine set in. This condition requires intense monitoring, and the problems resolve only after delivery.
- Combination hypertension. Some women with chronic hypertension may develop superimposed preeclampsia during pregnancy.

When blood pressure increases during pregnancy, it sometimes uncovers a tendency toward hypertension that may take years to evolve into a permanent elevation in blood pressure.

When blood pressure increases during pregnancy, it sometimes uncovers a tendency toward hypertension that may take years to evolve into a permanent elevation in blood pressure. This discovery can be a good thing. After all, most of us need some kind of motivation to do the things that Mom always told us to do—for example, eat right, get enough sleep, and exercise faithfully.

If your blood pressure was increased during pregnancy, you did not have preeclampsia, and your blood pressure has come down since concluding the pregnancy, you probably don't need blood pressure medicine right now; you just had gestational hypertension. Even so, it would be a good idea to keep periodic checks on your blood pressure, ideally at four- to six-month intervals. You don't need to see a doctor if you're able to check your blood pressure at home during this time. Gestational hypertension usually recurs at the next pregnancy, however, so you need to keep checking for high blood pressure during future pregnancies.

Unfortunately, research shows that women who demonstrate blood pressure increases during pregnancy are more prone to develop permanent hypertension later in life. One of the things we strive for is to discover hypertension as early as possible, and to treat it so that we maximally protect someone from the damage that prolonged high blood pressures (which have not been monitored) can cause.

16. Is anyone ever cured of hypertension?

Sometimes, but it's more the exception than the rule. We use the words "cure" and "hypertension" in the same sentence infrequently. People who have hypertension that is amenable to a cure typically have secondary hypertension (where the cause can be identified) or have experienced heart damage that renders the pump (i.e., the heart) incapable of sustaining the elevated blood pressure because of heart attack and/or heart failure.

People with curable hypertension tend to be younger and have a negative family history of hypertension. These criteria are not absolutes, but they are the common findings. Some causes of high blood pressure are quite dramatic, such as a tumor of the adrenal gland called a pheochromocytoma. This tumor makes enormous amounts of adrenaline, which it then releases randomly. Naturally, people with this kind of tumor

The first question that healthcare providers seek to answer when they see a patient with newly diagnosed hypertension is "Is the blood pressure increase in this person primary or secondary?"

Parenchymal

Pertaining to the pulp or tissue of an organ. It usually refers to the entire organ or tissue, and is used to distinguish the organ from its blood vessel or 'vascular' side. For example we use renal parenchymal disease to say the problem IS the whole kidney, and renal vascular disease when the problem is the blood supply TO the kidney.

---

are highly symptomatic, though the symptoms often crop up at unpredictable intervals. Adrenaline causes sweating, heart racing, and pounding headaches and can wreak havoc on your blood pressure. Removing this tumor can result in a dramatic improvement in symptoms and blood pressure. That's the good news. The *sobering* news is that only some 800 cases of this rare tumor occur each year in the United States. Consequently, looking for one is akin to searching for the proverbial needle in the haystack. When a pheochromocytoma is found and treated, however, improvements are usually dramatic.

This issue relates to the first question that a healthcare provider faces when evaluating a patient with hypertension: Is the hypertension primary or secondary? The goal of the physician is to find a secondary form whenever possible, because this diagnosis could mean sparing someone from lifelong antihypertensive drug therapy. However, some secondary forms of hypertension give us clues as to the cause but do not necessarily lead to a cure. One of the most common secondary causes of hypertension is impaired kidney function, called **parenchymal** kidney disease ("parenchymal" means the tissue itself). In fact, at least 90% of patients on dialysis—virtually all of whom have parenchymal kidney disease—have hypertension. In the period when their kidneys are failing, at least 80% of these individuals have hypertension, and yet there is no cure despite the clear connection between reduced kidney function and increased blood pressure levels. Put simply, secondary hypertension is not always curable. Nonetheless, healthcare providers still pursue identification of the secondary forms because it helps us to understand *why* someone's blood pressure is elevated even if we can't cure it. This information is also useful in choosing (and, in some cases, avoiding) blood pressure treatments.

Finally, most doctors' experience in managing patients with high blood pressure shows that some people experience episodes of prolonged blood pressure increases punctuated by periods during which their blood pressure falls back to normal levels. Said another way, hypertension appears to be close but is not sustained in some people. In my practice, when doing our three blood pressure checks over the course of a month, we sometimes find patients who demonstrate hypertension two out of three times and then are okay for a few visits, only to have their blood pressure increase yet again. In such cases, the lower blood pressure measurements aren't really the result of a cure, but rather indicate an exaggerated variability in the individual's blood pressure. For these patients, it's hard to know exactly when to start blood pressure medicines—that's why there's still an art aspect to medical care (as opposed to pure science). Part of the art lies in persuading patients to start taking medicines, and another part of the art is knowing when to have that discussion!

Virginia comments:

When I was diagnosed with hypertension, I remember feeling very much "over the hill" and I really minded "needing" medication for the first time in my life. The prospect of continuing the medication for the long term did not set too well either. I gradually accepted that these things were, in fact, true and that I needed to work with this problem just like the patients with whom I interacted. It was no longer "them" and "me" (the mindset that these things happen only to others), but "us."

17. What happens to my blood pressure when I am sleeping?

In a way, you could look at the time when you're asleep as a break for your circulation: Your activity is minimal, and as a result your metabolism needs are small. During this time, your circulation has a chance to have a breather. Your involuntary nervous system tends to be less active, you're not eating salt, and you typically are not facing stressful situations (unless that pepperoni pizza you had earlier in the evening is causing some real impressive dreamtime). Both the heart rate and the blood pressure tend to come down during the nighttime. We don't usually measure this decline outside of research settings, because we have not (at least not yet) shown that taking the nighttime blood pressure readings is important from a health perspective.

As mentioned in Question 11, some people are dippers (they experience a decrease in blood pressure during sleep) and some are non-dippers (they don't have this kind of blood pressure decrease). One of the values of exercise may be in that it promotes a dipper type of effect while a person is sleeping. By contrast, some of the damage to the heart and brain that occur in patients with kidney disease may reflect the fact that people with impaired kidney function are frequently non-dippers.

Whether and how much we dip seems to depend on the involuntary nervous system interaction while we are resting. Like most things in the body, there is a balance in the involuntary nervous system. This system consists of two parts. The **adrenergic** or **sympathetic** arm is the adrenaline-like side that speeds up your heart, increases your blood pressure, and gives you that "rush" feeling in exceptional circumstances. The **parasympathetic** side, which we understand less well, seems to slow heart rate and lower blood pressure. During sleep, the sympathetic nervous system yields the floor to the parasympathetic nervous system, so that heart rate slows and blood pressure falls. Somewhere in the wee hours of the morning, just before we get up, the sympathetic system takes back the reins and jump-starts the body with a shot of adrenaline to help us over that hump of facing the vertical position first thing in the morning. In some people, this activity contributes to heart attack and stroke, both of which occur more commonly in the first hours of the day and may be aided and abetted by the sympathetic surge.

Adrenergic

Related to adrenaline. The adrenergic portion of the involuntary nervous system is responsible for increasing heart rate and increasing blood pressure when stimulated.

Sympathetic

This term refers to that part of the involuntary nervous system that increase heart rate and increases blood pressure.

Parasympathetic

That part of the involuntary nervous system which balances the adrenaline or sympathetic effects. When the parasympathetic nervous system is active heart rates are slower and blood pressure is lower.

18. What should I know about my medical history to help my doctor take care of my hypertension?

If you are prepared to answer some questions about your medical history when you visit your doctor, you will help him or her more efficiently find the best way to evaluate and manage your high blood pressure. Some important items to know are whether other people in your family have hypertension, whether they take medication for it, and whether family members have experienced heart attacks or strokes and at what age. Also, can you recall the last time you know your blood pressure was normal? Are you taking blood pressure medicines now? If so, then it's a good idea to take the bottles with you so that the type, amount, and frequency of administration of your medication can be accurately recorded. Are you having any symptoms? If so, make a list of when they began, what time of day they occur, and how bothersome they are to you.

One of the most important issues is whether your high blood pressure has affected one of the target organs. As mentioned in Question 14, physicians evaluate patients with hypertension by asking three questions. The first question is whether the hypertension is primary or secondary; in secondary hypertension, the blood pressure increase is a symptom of another problem. A second question that physicians address when they see a new patient with elevated blood pressure is whether the hypertension has caused any harm to the patient. If you know you had a heart attack, angina, a previous stroke, circulation problems, heart failure, or damage to your kidneys, tell your doctor! It is important information to provide to your healthcare provider. Any details you can provide about these target organ problems will be very helpful. (We'll cover the third item in Question 22.)

Other things to discuss with your healthcare provider are medications you may have taken in the past. Did you find

Important items to know about your medical history are whether other people in your family have hypertension, whether they take medication for it, and whether family members have experienced heart attacks or strokes and at what age.

The second question that healthcare providers seek to answer when they see a patient with newly diagnosed hypertension is "Has the hypertension caused any harm to the patient?"

The Basics

some that you could not take because you felt bad or developed a problem such as a rash? It's very helpful to know the name of the medication that caused the problem.

Finally, it's very helpful to tell your healthcare provider whether you've had any kind of interventions in the past, such as a heart catheterization, an angioplasty, or a surgical procedure. If you want a gold star on this homework assignment, obtaining the records of these events will be of tremendous benefit to your physician.

19. At what age should my children have their blood pressure checked if I have hypertension?

You might not like the answer to this question: The pediatric associations recommend checking blood pressures for children as young as three years. Most pediatricians now do so, but it takes some special equipment because the blood pressure cuffs are smaller for such young children. Moreover, when it comes to hypertension in children, we don't use the same vocabulary as we do in adults. Instead, special tables are used to interpret blood pressure levels in children that are based on their gender and their height. At the end of this book, the resources list a Web site that you can access to see those tables. Many parents keep height and weight records for their children. It's not a bad idea to pencil in their blood pressures on this height or weight chart along with the little dot that we typically use to show their progress as they get older.

From a practical standpoint, elevated blood pressure that runs in families is difficult to detect as a really significant problem until a child reaches high school or college age. Not uncommonly, elevated blood pressures in children will be discovered when they try out for a sports team or some other school event that requires a physical examination. Nevertheless, some types of high blood pressure occur in children that are not necessarily linked to a family history. These conditions can be due to problems with the kidneys or other organs, so that the hypertension is actually a symptom of a different primary problem.

The moral of the story is that you are never really too young to start monitoring this important vital statistic. Hypertension often occurs with virtually no symptoms associated with it and is found only because someone took the time to check. To quote Yogi Berra, "You can see a lot by just looking."

20. Should I be lying down or sitting up when my blood pressure is taken?

In most people, the position during the blood pressure measurement will not make a huge difference in the reading. The most important thing is to have a five-minute rest before the actual blood pressure measurement is taken. (Have I said that before? See Question 8.) Nonetheless, one position does have an edge over the other. The correct answer to this question is "sitting." But why?

You might wonder why we treat high blood pressure with medicine at all. The answer is because it saves lives, reduces stroke, keeps hearts functioning well, and preserves kidney function. Of course, for many years high blood pressure was not treated with medicine. Beginning in the early 1960s, the first **clinical trials** of treatments for high blood pressure were undertaken and showed that there was benefit in lowering blood pressure with medications. How did the researchers who conducted these studies define someone as hypertensive, and how did they measure each participant's response to blood pressure medications over time? In most cases, they took the patient's blood pressure (usually several times) in a sitting position and used the same position subsequently to titrate blood pressure medication therapies.

How much difference is there in someone's blood pressure when taken in the supine (lying down) position compared

Clinical trials

This is considered the best way, or the "gold standard" to demonstrate the benefits of treatment. In a clinical trial a group of people with a finding (like hypertension) are randomly assigned one or another treatment (usually without the nature of the treatment being known to the doctors conducting the study or the patients taking the treatment: this is called "blinding") and followed for a long time to see if one treatment has better outcomes (like less strokes for example) compared with the other treatment.

to the sitting up position? Suppose you're lying down when your blood pressure is taken several times; these measurements average 144/92 mm Hg. When you sit up, the average is likely to be something like 140/94 mm Hg. That's a small difference—but remember that this value is an average. The top number tends to be a little lower on sitting up compared to lying down, and the lower number tends to be a little higher on sitting up compared with lying down.

In some people, the lower number goes up even more when they sit up compared to when they were lying down. The reason for the change is that the involuntary nervous system—in particular, the sympathetic part of it (see Question 17)— is charged with maintaining blood flow when you defy gravity. Lying down is the easiest position in which to deliver blood to the various organs. When you sit or stand, blood will prefer to pool, or collect, in your legs. To prevent that problem, the sympathetic nervous system leaps into action, so that the net result is a small fall in the upper number in the blood pressure reading and a small increase in the lower number. Some people have an exaggerated sympathetic nervous system response and will demonstrate bigger changes. For still other people, much less happens, so that sometimes there's no difference in the blood pressure measurements in the two positions.

To select the best therapy for you and achieve the results seen in medical research, it seems prudent to measure your blood pressure the same way the researchers did in the original clinical trials. For that reason, the sitting blood pressure is preferred. We still measure it lying down, and sometimes even standing up. Sometimes the changes seen in these positions can be quite dramatic, especially for the standing up blood pressure. This information is helpful to know because it can sometimes guide the choice of medicines that are used (or the choice of medicines that are discontinued) in individual patients whose blood pressure falls dramatically when they stand up.

21. I have headaches a lot. Are they caused by my high blood pressure?

The simple answer is they could be. People who suffer from migraine headaches, for example, clearly have changes in their blood vessels around the time that they experience headache pain. Moreover, in research studies of high blood pressure therapies, one of the side effects that appears consistently is headaches. The problem is that headaches are quite common. You may be having one now, which likely is related to muscle tension in the head area (and, of course, is not due to spending too much time reading this informative tome).

The kind of headaches that come specifically from hypertension are more commonly located in the back of the head, in an area called the **occiput.** When headaches occur in the front part of the head, and particularly when they affect only one side, we usually call them tension headaches. The same thing that causes tension also raises blood pressure, however, so a direct cause and effect of "blood pressure increase = headache" is often challenging to prove.

Occiput

The back part of the head or skull.

Despite this, it does seem that when people have headaches their blood pressures are higher. Another related finding is that pain increases blood pressure. In some ways, it's a "chicken and egg" problem: Did the increase in blood pressure cause the headache, or is the headache raising the blood pressure level? Often, the only way to determine the culprit is to take a medication that lowers blood pressure and see if the improvement in blood pressure control brings relief of the headache symptoms. Although I don't recommend this practice as a routine short-term undertaking, it is useful in some situations, especially when the blood pressure is very high.

One sign that headaches may follow from high blood pressure has to do with their presence when hypertension is newly diagnosed, and their subsequent disappearance after therapy is instituted and appears to be working. In that situation, it would appear that high blood pressure "causes" headaches.

One important, but rare circumstance in which headaches are clearly associated with blood pressure is a pheochromocytoma (see Question 16). This tumor, which affects the adrenal gland, makes its presence known by releasing significant amounts of adrenaline. The headaches associated with a pheochromocytoma are very much like migraines in that they are pounding, episodic, and often associated with a racing heart. This is one situation where it's very important to make your healthcare provider aware of your headache story. Pheochromocytoma is one of the few kinds of high blood pressure where we do, indeed, use the word "cure" in the same sentence with "hypertension": Surgical removal of these tumors usually cures the headaches and the hypertension.

22. Is there a blood test or a gene test that can tell whether someone will develop high blood pressure someday?

There is no dearth of effort to find this magic bullet that will predict accurately who will develop hypertension someday. In some very rare cases, syndromes of high blood pressure stem from a single defect in a single gene. These kind of defects, as a group, probably explain less than 1% of all hypertension, however. Scientists tend to think that hypertension results from many gene defects, not just one. Moreover, in addition to the genetic issues, environmental influences probably promote the development of hypertension.

Genetic testing is not frequently done in hypertension care, and no blood test can predict the onset of hypertension.

Sometimes, people have a phenotype in which hypertension is part of the story. A phenotype is an appearance or certain "look" about a person. If you've ever seen the movie *The Elephant Man,* then you know that this patient had a very characteristic appearance. It turns out that the syndrome that afflicted John Merrick, called neurofibromatosis, is associated with high blood pressure. So are a handful of other disorders, such as von Hippel Lindau disease. Thus it's not always necessary to do a genetic test—sometimes you can predict the development of hypertension with high likelihood based on someone's appearance or the fact that he or she has a family history of a particular syndrome.

Genetic testing is not frequently done in hypertension care. We do, however, know that certain rare tumors, such as pheochromocytoma and its cousin paraganglioma, often have gene mutations associated with them. When someone has one of these kinds of tumors, healthcare providers usually recommend genetic testing for both the patient and his or her children. In some cases, the types of genetic testing can also help predict which of these tumors are more likely to behave in a malignant fashion.

There is no blood test that can predict the onset of hypertension. Even so, we can measure many components in the blood for which abnormal levels are associated with high blood pressure. We called these findings in the blood **biomarkers.** One such biomarker was mentioned in Question 7—namely, cholesterol. Potential biomarkers of hypertension include blood sugar, insulin level, the triglyceride concentration, and markers of **inflammation** such as high-sensitivity C-reactive protein (hs-CRP); their levels are frequently in the "bad" range in people with hypertension.

Remember the three issues or questions that physicians address when evaluating a patient with hypertension? (See Question 14.) Our current discussion brings us to the third one: the search for **cardiovascular** risk factors that, in conjunction with hypertension, put someone at higher likelihood for having heart disease or stroke in the future. Although the blood tests mentioned previously do not predict hypertension, we measure them anyway because they help us understand the amount of risk for any one hypertensive person. We'll cover this issue in more detail in later questions.

The Basics

Biomarkers

A term applied to things we measure in the blood or urine that have relevance (good or bad) to disease. Some are hormones, some are proteins, and some are just small molecules that accumulate, or are depleted, in specific disease states. For example the good form of cholesterol, 'HDL-cholesterol', is a biomarker. See question 22 for others.

Inflammation

This term refers to the ability of a hormone, or a germ like a bacteria or virus, or some other influence to cause a reaction in the body that involves some aspect of the immune system. The result of this reaction is often a build up of scar or plaque. Inflammation is thought to play a big role in hardening of the arteries.

Cardiovascular

Relating to the heart or blood vessels.

PART TWO

Lifestyle and Exercise

What kinds of lifestyle changes do I need to make if
I have hypertension?

Why does additional weight seem to cause my blood
pressure to go up?

If I lose weight, will my blood pressure improve and
by how much?

More . . .

23. What kinds of lifestyle changes do I need to make if I have hypertension?

A person can take four steps to manage his or her blood pressure short of taking pressure-lowering medications:

- Lose weight if you are overweight.
- Reduce your salt intake.
- Get some exercise.
- Limit your daily alcohol intake to three drinks if you are male, and to two drinks if you are female.

As a practical matter, each time you lose about 2 pounds, you will drop approximately one point (1 mm Hg) on the blood pressure scale. For example, the loss of 20 pounds could lead to as much as a 10 mm Hg drop in your blood pressure readings. Of course, this precise result isn't guaranteed, because this information came from studying large groups of people, not particular individuals. Nevertheless, weight loss offers several benefits beside better blood pressure control, including better lipid levels, breathing easier when climbing steps, and a longer time before you have to consider joint replacement of your knees for starters.

The issues with salt are relatively complicated. Only one-half to two-thirds of patients with high blood pressure are salt-sensitive: They experience a lowering of blood pressure when they reduce their salt intake. Unfortunately, that means one-third to one-half of patients with high blood pressure are salt-resistant: They *don't* have blood pressure changes when they reduce their salt intake. We don't have infallible ways of measuring a person's salt sensitivity with respect to his or her blood pressure, so we rely on common findings from studies conducted in this area to predict whether someone is likely to benefit from salt reduction. As a rule of thumb, people of African American ethnicity, people older than age 60, people who are overweight, and people with diabetes and kidney failure are more likely to be salt-sensitive.

One of my friends described exercise as "running when no one is chasing you, and lifting things that do not really need to be moved." Many of us undoubtedly share his cynical attitude toward exercise. But exercise certainly has some good aspects, and you don't have to spend an hour each day in intensity aerobic activity to get some benefit from it. Actually, 20–30 minutes of brisk walking performed daily would do all of us a lot of good. Even this kind of moderate exercise tends to have a modest effect on lowering blood pressure, and it also helps blunt the appetite. Furthermore, it can improve lipid metabolism by lowering triglyceride levels and increasing the good form of cholesterol, known as **high-density lipoprotein (HDL) cholesterol.** Moreover, regular exercise, particular in conjunction with weight loss, can reduce your chance of developing diabetes someday.

Lastly, we come to our old friend John Barleycorn (i.e., alcohol, in all its many forms). It's difficult to put alcohol intake into perspective when it comes to overall cardiovascular risk management. The advice of the Canadian "Jack Rabbit" Johansen (who introduced cross-country skiing to North America) may be best here. When he was asked how he lived so long (he was about 90 years old at the time), he replied, "Don't drink too much, . . . and then again don't drink too little." If you are a teetotaler, you won't obtain any blood-pressure-reducing benefit by suddenly starting to consume one or two drinks a day. Conversely, you can expect some blood pressure improvement if you regularly have more than three drinks per day on average, and cut back to less than three drinks per day.

Virginia comments:

This is the part of treatment that takes most of my time and effort. Dr T. explained very well the changes needed, but, even though most of us understand the facts, the results of research findings, the benefits these changes could make, even the extension of our lives, and so on, we all know how difficult actually making these changes

High-density lipoprotein (HDL) cholesterol

High-density lipoprotein cholesterol; also called the 'good' cholesterol. HDL cholesterol is thought to return cholesterol from places like blood vessel linings to the liver for excretion in the bile.

really is! Of all people, I should weigh in within the normal weight range for my age and height. Alas, I haven't seen that weight for some years. The middle years of my life were fraught with the complexities of teen-aged kids acting up, financial strain, going back to school for an advanced degree, a full-time job, aging ill parents, and, well, you get the idea! Now that I am in my sixties, I find my weight is gradually creeping back to the normal range—probably because my lifestyle has been simplified and I have more energy for exercise and meal planning, plus I indulge in much less "emotional eating" (when we eat even though we are not hungry).

I would encourage those readers who find themselves in the throes of stress and problems to seek the support of professionals for weight loss, anxiety, smoking cessation, marital difficulties, assistance caring for aging parents, or whatever other stressors may be barriers to your good health. Support and validation for your unique life situation are invaluable.

24. Why does additional weight seem to cause my blood pressure to go up?

Our understanding of what fat cells do has changed dramatically in the past 20 years. We used to think these cells just sat there storing fat, then released their fat supplies once in a while when energy demands were high and carbohydrate availability was low. Now we realize that fat cells are incredibly active, and that they make all sorts of hormones that can affect blood pressure. Consequently, when more fat cells are present or when the average fat cell is bigger, the body's hormone production tends to increase.

Angiotensinogen

A protein made by the liver and to a lesser extent the fat cells. This protein is ultimately metabolized by enzymes to yield angiotensin-II a very potent blood pressure raising hormone.

Some of these hormones are quite beneficial. For example, fat cells make adiponectin, a hormone that helps insulin work better at keeping the blood sugar in line. Unfortunately, fat cells also make several chemicals that directly raise blood pressure, such as **angiotensinogen.** Perhaps you've heard of drugs called angiotensin-converting enzyme (ACE) inhibitors? These medications lower blood pressure by directly interfering with the metabolism of angiotensinogen. Moreover, several **inflammatory** biomarkers (see Question 22) come from fat cells. These inflammatory biomarkers are thought to participate in **atherosclerosis,** or hardening of the arteries. As a result of the **atherosclerotic** process, arteries become stiffer, which can in turn raise your blood pressure—especially the upper blood pressure number.

Another problem with weight gain is that it can predispose you to the development of diabetes. Diabetes and hypertension are like the gangsters Bonnie and Clyde: Each is bad enough when alone, but put them together and trouble is sure to follow. The presence of diabetes doubles your risk of eventually developing hypertension; the presence of hypertension doubles your risk of eventually developing diabetes. The last couple of decades have witnessed a progressive increase in the average weight of adults in the United States, and this increase in weight has been matched step-by-step by an increase in the prevalence of diabetes. Consequently, one of your best hedges against someday developing diabetes is to keep your weight down. Question 23 offers some pointers for how to do so. When a person has both diabetes and hypertension, his or her cardiovascular risk is relatively serious, so avoid this combination if you can.

25. If I lose weight, will my blood pressure improve and by how much?

Question 23 described the blood pressure benefit from losing weight. Typically, losing 2 pounds brings a 1 mm Hg decrease in blood pressure. This decline in blood pressure does not go on indefinitely, however. For example, losing 100 pounds is unlikely to lead to a 50-point drop in your blood pressure. The good news is you don't have to lose all 100 pounds to get the blood pressure benefit. Most of the improvements will occur after you lose the first 20 to 30 pounds.

Inflammatory

This term refers to the ability of a hormone, or a germ like a bacteria or virus, or some other influence to cause a reaction in the body that involves some aspect of the immune system. The result of this reaction is often a build up of scar or plaque. Inflammation is thought to play a big role in hardening of the arteries.

Atherosclerosis & atherosclerotic

These terms refer to hardening of the artery usually from the build up of cholesterol plaque in the innermost lining of a vessel which can limit or block blood flow in that vessel.

When a person has both diabetes and hypertension, his or her cardiovascular risk is relatively serious, so avoid this combination if you can.

In addition, the means by which you lose weight can influence how much blood pressure benefit you experience. There are at least three ways to lose weight.

First, you can alter your diet and exercise patterns. You could starve, of course, but the better approach is to make a conscious effort to reduce your calorie intake, which is more sensible but works a bit more slowly. There is no dearth of books on how to achieve this goal—several are collecting dust on the bookshelf somewhere in my office at this very moment. Both the South Beach diet and the Atkins diet seem to work fairly well when followed conscientiously. The latest craze is the Dash diet (see the "Literature and Other Sources of Information" appendix at the end of this book for Web site information).

If you've ever taken a course in physics, you are familiar with the law of conservation of energy: "Energy cannot be created or destroyed, but can only be changed from one form to another." This means that if you eat 100 calories and expend 90 of them through exercise, the other 10 calories don't just go away. Instead, they change from one form (for example, a potato chip) to another form—specifically, fat. Each 3000 to 3500 calories that we eat in excess of our body's need for energy ends up being stored as about a pound of fat. In other words, we have to burn this many calories in excess of what we take if we want to lose a pound of fat. This "road to a thinner you" can seem daunting when you do the math. In my practice, I tell patients that it took a long time to build up the weight and it will take a while to lose it (at least when it comes to the dietary deprivation method). My usual goal is to get people to lose about 4 to 6 pounds per month. If they achieve that goal, then I'm thrilled.

The second way to lose weight is to think of DuPont's slogan: "Better living through chemistry." Several medications are available that can assist people in losing weight. These drugs tend to work by either blocking fat absorption in the intestine or trying to speed up metabolism of calories through the sympathetic nervous system. The problem with the latter approach is that it can sometimes raise (rather than lower) blood pressure because part of its mechanism of action is to mimic the sympathetic nervous system (see Question 17). In general, people tend to lose 10 to 15 pounds in the first six months when treated with medicines, but then things get kind of stagnant. Moreover, once they stop taking the medicines, many people tend to regain the lost weight because they don't eat any differently. Although physicians sometimes prescribe these medicines to their overweight patients who have hypertension, we often do so hoping that better alternatives will become available in future. One auspicious compound is a new drug that is now available in Europe called rimonabant. This medicine has had good success in spurring weight loss, but the evidence so far suggests that its use provides only a small benefit in terms of lowering blood pressure.

The third way—and one of the most effective ways—to lose weight, and lose it quickly, is to have a **bariatric** surgical procedure. This procedure could involve either banding the stomach (gastric banding) or undergoing a gastrointestinal bypass. People who undergo such procedures typically lose 70 pounds or more in the course of the year after surgery. Moreover, the weight does tend to stay off, though these procedures are usually reserved for people who are really large and have failed to lose weight with either dietary restrictions or weight loss medications. Although bariatric procedures are a drastic way to lose weight, they are growing in popularity—in part because the number of people who are truly obese is also growing. Although this strategy is quite effective in terms of producing weight loss, we're still waiting to see what the long-term consequences of this kind of approach to weight control might be.

Bariatric
Pertaining to weight.

26. How does too much salt cause my blood pressure to increase?

In people who are salt-sensitive, the ingestion of salt contributes to blood pressure increase two ways:

- Through **cardiac output**
- Through the interaction of salt intake with hormones that raise blood pressure

Cardiac output

The quantity of blood, usually expressed in liters/minute, pumped by the heart each minute.

Cardiac output refers to how much blood the heart pumps per minute. A typical value is about 6 quarts per minute (roughly 6 liters per minute). When we take in salt, we actually expand the blood volume, which in turn increases the cardiac output. In people who are salt-resistant, the body adjusts its blood flow "spigots" (i.e., the resistance—see Question 2) by opening them up a little bit to accommodate the increase in cardiac output so that the blood pressure doesn't actually rise. In people who are salt-sensitive, the body does not adjust the spigots; thus, when the cardiac output increases, the blood pressure rises along with it.

Several hormones play important roles in controlling the blood pressure. Angiotensinogen (see Question 24), for example, is converted to angiotensin II, which then raises blood pressure. The combination of salt intake and angiotensin II causes the blood pressure to increase even more dramatically than it would have owing to the effects of the angiotensin II alone. The same is true for adrenaline. Salt acts like gasoline poured on a fire when it comes to blood pressure in salt-sensitive patients. In essence, it tends to partner with other chemicals that raise blood pressure and amplifies their effects.

How much salt is safe? According to the American Heart Association, the maximum amount is 2400 mg of sodium per day. When you look at food labels and tally up their sodium content, that's the number to shoot for. Sodium, however, is only half of the team we call "salt"; the other half is the compound called chloride. It turns out that most sodium is partnered with chloride; consequently, when you tote up the amount of sodium, you're basically figuring out the amount of chloride present as well. Every 2000 mg of added dietary sodium you consume probably contributes 2 or 3 mm Hg to your blood pressure.

Here are some simple rules to help you cut down on your salt intake:

- The most effective strategy is to eat your meals at home or at least to prepare them at your home. In the latter case, that means making your lunch yourself, and not letting the fast-food places do the cooking for you (at least not most of the time).
- Put the salt shaker away, mail it to your aunt in Toledo, give it away as a freebie at your next garage sale, or otherwise get rid of it. In this case, the old adage "Out of sight, out of mind" is definitely a good thing.
- Reduce your intake of preprocessed foods. Part of the preservation of foods involves putting salt in the food product. Keep in mind the big offenders when it comes to salt intake: soups, lunch meats, dairy products (particularly cheese), chips, pretzels, ice cream, and certain vegetable juices such as V8 and tomato juice (read the labels to be sure).

27. Is it okay to use Morton's Lite-Salt or sea salt?

Morton's Lite Salt is a combination of sodium chloride and potassium chloride. Consumption of potassium is generally safe, as long as you don't take other medicines that are adversely affected by it. These medications include potassium-sparing **diuretics** such as spironolactone, amiloride, and triamterene, which often appear in combination in the same tablet or capsule with hydrochlorothiazide (HCTZ). Some people are also sensitive to potassium intake when they use

Diuretic

Substance or medication that causes an increase in urine excretion. Caffeine is an example of a naturally occurring mild diuretic. Hydrochlorothiazide, or HCTZ, is an example of a prescription diuretic.

certain pain relievers, such as ibuprofen. Likewise, people with kidney failure are prone to potassium-related problems, so it's not a good idea to take extra potassium when your kidneys are not working well without checking with your doctor first. If you're not on these medicines and your kidney function is normal, then an occasional sprinkle (not a liberal application) of Morton's Light Salt is probably okay and better than using the straight salt shaker.

Sea salt is salt. It may sound kind of healthy but it's still salt. See Question 26.

28. How does stress affect my blood pressure, and by how much?

We do not fully understand the relationship between stress and hypertension, but we have a few tentative answers to this question. What has hampered research in this area is the lack of a stress unit. When we measure blood pressure, we get values like 140/84 mm Hg. In this case, the unit "mm Hg" is something we can describe and quantify; it is an objective measure. It's not as possible to do the same thing with stress, because the effects of stressful situations are not felt the same way by each person who experiences them—some people tend to be more reactive than others. We measure stress with relative scales (i.e., subjective measures) where you might make a mark on a line closer to one side than the other to indicate how stressed you are feeling on a scale of 1 to 5 or 1 to 10, as in **Figure 3.**

Researchers have made an effort to find quantifiable, objective measures of stress in the body. For example, we know that stress tends to increase the amounts of two important chemicals in the body: adrenaline and **cortisol.** Adrenaline is a great way to "electrify" the circulation. It makes the heart pump faster and harder, and it typically raises the blood pressure. Cortisol functions like the body's aspirin. It has anti-inflammatory effects, and it can relieve pain (as people with

Cortisol

A hormone from the cortex of the adrenal gland which is produced to offset inflammation in the body.

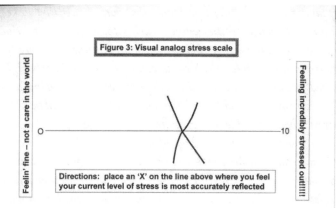

Figure 3   Visual Analog Stress Scale

rheumatoid arthritis are well aware, because cortisol helps diminish their arthritic flares). Unfortunately, cortisol also works to conserve salt in the body by reducing its losses in the urine. In addition, cortisol has other, less well understood effects that result in raised blood pressure.

How much effect stress has on blood pressure has been widely debated. If we measure blood pressure carefully in air-traffic controllers at their worksite, the readings tend to be higher there than those taken at home. Likewise, blood pressure measurements in controllers taken at their worksite are higher compared with blood pressure measurements for people who work in a relaxed office setting where there is less hazard associated with their jobs. Even so, it is very hard to put a precise number on how much stress affects any one person's blood pressure.

Virginia comments:

This question is often answered by the 24-hour ambulatory blood pressure monitor (ABPM). In my case, I lectured to the nursing school about hypertension. Part of the lecture involved my wearing and explaining the function of the ABPM. I also learned the heights to which my blood pressure would go during public

It is very hard to put a precise number on how much stress affects any one person's blood pressure.

speaking (scary). I asked patients who wore the ABPM to keep a diary of their activities while wearing the monitor. Situations such as business meetings, being late for an appointment, any type of argument, even telephone calls, would produce noticeably higher blood pressures. I once asked a college professor if lecturing made him nervous. He said he had been doing it for years and he felt no stress whatsoever. He was very surprised when he saw his ABPM report, which showed very high blood pressures during the lecture. Clearly, many times people are not even aware of their stressors. Sometimes we can institute measures to avoid these episodes, such as leaving earlier for appointments so that a traffic jam is not so upsetting, learning meditative skills, and so on.

29. If I am diagnosed with hypertension, does that mean that I shouldn't exercise?

You don't need to spend hours and hours in the gym to experience a benefit from exercise. One of the best exercises is a brisk walk.

When people have newly diagnosed hypertension and their blood pressure values are really high, then they should probably refrain from exercise. Until their blood pressure decreases to a much more manageable level by virtue of therapy, it probably isn't wise to exercise. However, once their blood pressure starts to come under control with medication, it is usually safe to commence an exercise program at that point. As mentioned previously, you don't need to spend hours and hours in the gym to experience a benefit. One of the best exercises is a brisk walk because it moves some of the largest muscle groups (your legs) and both consumes energy (so it helps you to maintain or lose weight) and reduces your blood pressure.

Given the ease with which your blood pressure can be measured in many different settings, including the gym as well as your home, you can take the guesswork out of what kind of response you're having during and after exercise by actually measuring your blood pressure. This kind of monitoring violates one of my commandments about blood pressure measurement (see Question 8). Even so, it is important—for example, in cardiac rehabilitation programs—to monitor the blood pressure changes that someone experiences while walking or doing some other kind of exercise, particularly if the person has experienced heart damage in the past.

If your heart's okay as far you know, but you happen to be a 50-year-old smoker with hypertension and a worrisome **lipid profile** (for example, a high cholesterol level), you should talk with your healthcare provider before buying an LA Fitness subscription and going at it with a passion. Sometimes, we will put someone through an exercise stress test when they have worrisome cardiovascular risk factors and want to exercise even if they are without symptoms. Although it isn't a perfect screening test, such a test does make sense for some people.

> **Lipid profile**
>
> A blood test, usually done after fasting for 8 or more hours, that measures cholesterol (total, good and bad forms) and triglycerides levels.

30. How will I know how much exercise is safe?

There are a few things you can do to ensure your safety when it comes to exercise. The most obvious measures are common sense. If you find yourself remarkably short of breath or developing chest discomfort with moderate activity levels, then slow down. If you find yourself breaking into a vigorous sweat, reconsider your activity level. If you're lightheaded, you may be doing too much. If your blood pressure rises to more than 200 mm Hg during activity, then the exercise may cause problems for you.

It's not easy to know what a "safe" level of exercise is in any particular individual. Although we know hypertension has long-term risks, it's very hard to predict what short-term increases in blood pressure mean in an individual.

If you have any issues with respect to heart disease, stroke, or peripheral circulation problems, it makes sense to check your blood pressures frequently when you're participating in an exercise program. You can do this kind of monitoring yourself, or site personnel may be already trained to do this very thing if you go to a dedicated area. In any of these circumstances, having a heart-to-heart talk with your healthcare provider is a good idea before you invest in your next pair of expensive running shoes.

31. Is it true that I should not lift weights if I have hypertension?

The answer to this question is both yes and no. There are at least two kinds of weight lifting, and the type you pursue determines the answer for you.

One kind of weight lifting involves lifting incredibly large amounts of weight (with the attendant grunts and groans) and holding the mass of metal above your head until someone brings a bell and announces "Winner." This practice, which is called bench pressing or lifting, can be bad for the heart. At the time when your muscles are straining to hold this huge weight above your body, your blood pressure can be off the charts in your arms, and your heart is hard pressed to pump blood through your muscles during this time. The result is some thickening in the heart muscle, which can lead to problems later on. Bench pressing can also raise your systolic blood pressure even after you drop the weight and walk away with your trophy. One lingering concern is that some people who do this kind of lifting also take anabolic steroids to aid in their muscle development. Anabolic steroids will also raise your blood pressure.

The alternative to bench pressing is repetitive lighter-weight lifts, or reps for short. Unlike the sustained lifting found in bench pressing, reps entail short repeated cycles where muscles stretch, relax, and stretch again. This is a much "friendlier" type of exercise when it comes to blood pressure, and physicians tend to encourage people who want to lift weights to do it this way, and discourage those who seek to develop the upper torso of Rocky Balboa through the previously mentioned lifting activities.

32. Will jogging or running put too much strain on my heart?

The answer to this question depends on several factors, such as how old you are, how high your blood pressure is, and whether you have any evidence of circulation problems at this time. If you're 25 and hypertensive, odds are that you can jog or run and you'll be fine. If you're 65 and working on your third bypass procedure, it is a different story. If your blood pressure is uncontrolled, it's a good idea to wait until it is controlled with medication before commencing or restarting a jogging or running program.

Those of us who don't jog or run sometimes have a hard time understanding why others do. In general, in the absence of known heart disease (or problems such as knee cartilage damage), jogging and running are fine exercises. In my practice, I have cared for people who continued to jog up to the age of 65 or 70 years and who played singles tennis several times a week. The issue here is one of common sense. Listen to your body: It will usually tell you when you need to slow down.

Listen to your body: It will usually tell you when you need to slow down.

33. If I perspire while exercising, could my blood pressure go down too much?

The amount of salt and water you lose through sweat, even when you exercise quite vigorously, is relatively small compared to the circulating blood volume. Consequently, your blood pressure is unlikely to go down very much just from sweating unless you are really overdoing matters. Nevertheless, there are a few important things to keep in mind with respect to this issue.

First, some people take medications that might exacerbate sweat-associated losses of salt water. For example, diuretics work by depleting the body of salt, so the additional loss through perspiration could add up in a person who takes a diuretic medication. You'll know that your blood pressure is drifting down if you feel lightheaded or dizzy.

The second circumstance is more subtle. It tends to occur in older people who are out in the sun for a prolonged period of time, such as while gardening. Older people have fewer defenses against the losses of salt water through the skin and are more prone to blood pooling in the lower extremities. Thus they are more prone to having symptoms as a consequence of perspiration loss, especially when getting up from a squatting position after gardening for a while on a hot July day.

Generally there is no benefit but some potential harm in taking salt tablets before you exercise. Fortunately, this practice has become much less frequent now than it was 20 or 30 years ago. The sensible thing to do is to be sure you're adequately hydrated before you exercise. This will give you a little reserve in terms of fluids.

34. By how much can regular exercise lower my blood pressure?

You can expect a 4 to 6 mm Hg reduction, on average, in your blood pressure as a consequence of an exercise program.

One of the best times to check your blood pressure is about 15 to 20 minutes after you take a good walk or engage in a workout in the gym. These are likely to be the best blood pressure values you'll see in any 24-hour period. According to the major guidelines for managing hypertension, which are called the Joint National Committee's reports (see the end of this book for the Web site), you can expect a 4 to 6 mm Hg reduction, on average, in your blood pressure as a consequence of an exercise program.

That's the good news. The bad news is that exercise works only when you exercise. If you give up exercising, you tend to lose the benefits to your blood pressure that the exercise provided over the next one to two months. Interestingly, the benefits of exercise on blood pressure know no age limits. In other words, the excuse, "I'm too old to be doing that," just doesn't hold water in this instance.

35. If I exercise regularly, can I stop my medication?

Not without a note from your doctor. Most of the effects of lifestyle changes on your blood pressure are smaller in magnitude than the effects associated with the blood pressure medicine. If someone begins exercising when he or she previously was sedentary and sees a nice blood pressure response, it's natural to wonder, "Why can't I chuck that medicine out the window and just do this exercise thing instead?"

Once in a while, it is possible to taper and discontinue medication in someone who successfully achieves lifestyle changes in a bid to control his or her blood pressure. This kind of case, however, tends to be more the exception than the rule. In general, lifestyle changes are complementary to blood pressure medication. However, if you can get your blood pressure consistently down to the range of 120/80 mm Hg and you're taking just one blood pressure medication, then you might be able to sustain your blood pressure in the nonhypertensive range even if you were to reduce or discontinue your medication. In my practice, I'm more likely to suggest a drug holiday when someone has blood pressures that are on the low side following lifestyle changes, but only if the person is willing to monitor his or her blood pressures at home after drug reduction or discontinuation.

Medical research studies support the idea that some people can safely discontinue their medications when they make these kinds of lifestyle changes. Unfortunately, many of these individuals will experience a resurgence of their blood pressure over time, which is why it's so important to carefully monitor blood pressures if medication is stopped. It's always advisable to have your healthcare provider participate in this decision-making process. Sometimes, medicines that are used for blood pressure control have other benefits. Members of the drug class called beta blockers, for example, not only lower blood pressure, but also treat certain heart disorders such as angina and heart failure. You might find that while you think the medication was used for lowering your blood pressure, your doctor thinks that it was treating your blood pressure *and* something else. That possibility is one of many reasons why it's a good idea to have your doctor be involved in decisions about your medications.

36. How, exactly, does exercise help blood pressure?

Several systems, known collectively as servos, help to maintain our blood pressure. One particularly important system is called the baroreceptor system. The prefix *baro* means "pressure," and *receptor* means "something that senses." In English, then, the baroreceptor senses the blood pressure level. When the blood pressure falls, the baroreceptor reacts to that event by increasing the heart rate and the sympathetic nervous system action so that blood vessels squeeze and narrow (constrict) and blood pressure is maintained. Somewhere along the way, the baroreceptor has to decide where its baseline should be. One theory about the origins of high blood pressure is that hypertension occurs in part because the baroreceptor resets at a higher level and defends that higher level of blood pressure, which is now in the greater than 140/90 mm Hg range. Among other things, exercise appears to reset the baroreceptor to a lower, healthier level.

Insulin resistance

A situation in which insulin has difficulty promoting sugar uptake into body cells (the cells are resistant). High levels of insulin and sometimes blood sugar results. People with insulin resistance are higher risk for developing diabetes.

Exercise also helps in producing and maintaining weight loss. As mentioned previously, weight and blood pressure are clearly related. Part of the benefit of exercise on blood pressure is, therefore, mediated through weight loss.

Finally, exercise appears to improve the way insulin (a hormone) acts to control blood sugar. We call this phenomenon insulin sensitivity. People who are **insulin resistant** require higher levels of insulin to keep their blood sugar under control. One potential consequence associated with this kind of insulin resistance is hypertension. When a person exercises regularly, insulin sensitivity tends to improve. In fact, people who are insulin resistant tend to become less insulin resistant when they exercise. This explains why exercise can help prevent diabetes. When people are more insulin sensitive, their circulation tends to be better behaved and they have less hypertension.

37. I have arthritis. Does that mean I can't exercise?

If the arthritis is truly extensive, then the answer to this question may be "Yes, the pain you would experience from the exercise would trump any benefit on your blood pressure." However, many people with arthritis can engage in at least some kind of exercise, especially given their creative nature, which enables many of them to find ways to do things despite their handicaps. For example, water aerobics is often a possibility, and there are lots of exercises other than walking that people can do. Moreover, rheumatologists tend to believe that exercise is actually fairly healthy for joints, even achy ones.

Unfortunately, some of the medications that people take for arthritis can work against their blood pressure. If you take these kinds of pain relievers, you may have gotten notes from your pharmacist that read like something out of a Stephen King novel, filled with all sorts of dire warnings about high blood pressure, heart attack, and other circulatory disorders. It is true that some antiarthritis medications will raise blood pressure. If anything, this relationship suggests that it is potentially useful to exercise in an effort to offset some of the effects of these medicines on the blood pressure.

Is there anyone who will not benefit from exercise or—worse yet—might be harmed by it? The answer is yes. The American Heart Association has identified at least two circumstances in which exercise could be harmful or is at least *not* helpful (*Circulation* 2007;115:2358–2368):

Hypertrophic cardiomyopathy

Cardiomyopathy is a condition in which the muscle of the heart is abnormal in the absence of an apparent cause.

- **Hypertrophic cardiomyopathy.** This rare hereditary disorder of thickened heart muscle sometimes causes relatively young people to drop dead while exercising. Thicker heart muscle behaves differently than regular heart muscle, and is more prone to skipping or stopping. Hypertrophic cardiomyopathy is typically diagnosed by echocardiogram (see the glossary for more information).

Anomalous coronary arteries

The term coronary artery anomaly refers to a wide range of congenital abnormalities involving the origin, course, and structure of epicardial coronary arteries.

- **Anomalous coronary arteries.** In this condition, the coronary arteries (the blood vessels that supply blood to the heart itself) arise from places other than their usual origin right at the beginning of the aorta. Because they arise from an anomalous ("weird") place, they may not be able to supply the additional blood the heart needs when exercising, unlike normal coronary arteries. (See the glossary for more information.)

38. Now that I have been diagnosed with hypertension, should I join a gym immediately?

The answer to this question will depend on your degree of motivation. If you're the kind of person who feels extreme guilt about spending money on a gym membership and not using it, then perhaps that tactic will get you inside the doors. The real key is not so much the venue in which you exercise, but your willingness to *actually* exercise—period. If you live at the North Pole, your chances of comfortably walking one to two miles per day in a short-sleeve shirt at a modest clip are marginal. For the rest of us who live in more southerly climates, much of the year we can be outside enjoying nature while burning a few calories and improving our **vascular** health.

Vascular

This term refers to blood vessels. It usually, but not always, refers to the artery type of blood vessels in particular.

Many organizations are actively promoting the idea of more Americans getting more exercise. Question 37 mentioned the American Heart Association's recent statement on exercise. You might also have seen the public-service announcements on television that recommend picking up the pace when you walk from one place to another. The goal here is not to become a world-class athlete with superb cardiovascular conditioning and a heart rate similar to that of a sea turtle. Much more modest goals are what we are after—specifically, trying to get 20–30 minutes of quality walking time in per day. In my opinion, the best use of your time for exercise is time devoted to this kind of exercise. Many patients report that "I do lots of walking at my job." Even so, the benefits of walking seemed to be a bit more likely to accrue when you exercise without a deadline in mind, and without the duress of the workplace.

When I took my current job, I made a mental commitment to walk from the train station to my workplace, which takes 15 to 20 minutes. In my mind, that trip counts as exercise. There are lots of clever ways to engage in some extra walking to the workplace, from the workplace, or even for errands. Although walking is not the only form of exercise, of course, it tends to be one of the easiest to do. At the same time, there's nothing wrong—and perhaps something desirable—with joining a gym and selecting a workout regimen that's tailored to your particular needs. Most gyms have staff members who will be glad to help you in this regard. The advice of the sneaker company Nike is probably relevant here: "Just do it."

39. I have heard that people who do not breathe well when sleeping have more heart problems. Is this related to blood pressure?

This comment refers to the phenomenon known as sleep disordered breathing, also called sleep apnea. People with this condition have loud snoring, gasping, and periods of time when they do not seem to be moving air even though they appear to be trying to breathe while sleeping. They often wake up short of breath either because their brain tells them, "Wake up and breathe," or because their bed partner shakes them awake and says, "You weren't breathing."

These periods of poor breathing reduce the amount of oxygen available, and the brain reacts to this message with panic. Part of the panic response includes an increase in heart rate and an increase in blood pressure. Does that sound familiar? These signs indicate that the sympathetic nervous system is active. When we measure the activity of this branch of the nervous system (for example, by measuring adrenaline excretion), it tends to go up during these periods. These little bouts of increased heart rate and blood pressure take their toll on the heart itself and on the circulation in general. A recent study called the Sleep Heart Health Study revealed that there are more cardiovascular outcomes (such as heart attack and heart failure) in people who have this kind of sleep apnea. (See the "Literature and Other Sources of Information" appendix for more information on the Sleep Heart Health Study.)

Sleep disordered breathing is diagnosed through a sleep study, also known as a polysomnogram (PSG). In this kind of study, you are wired up, a blood pressure cuff is fitted to your arm, an oxygen sensor is fitted to your finger or some other place, and little electrodes are placed in various locations on your body. Once you are maximally uncomfortable (just kidding), the technician will smile and tell you, "Okay, now it's time to go to sleep." Surprisingly enough, many people are able to sleep despite all these trappings. During the time that you sleep, the various recording devices note your respiration, heart rate, blood pressure, and oxygen levels.

When the sleep study confirms that a person has sleep apnea, your doctor will usually discuss options for handling this situation. One of the most common treatments involves a continuous positive airway pressure (CPAP) device. You can't miss people using CPAP—they look like they belong in the cockpit of an F-16 fighter plane. A tightly fitting mask is crafted to their face, and a certain degree of airway pressure is maintained while they're sleeping so that their airway doesn't collapse. Research is now under way to determine just how much benefit CPAP has for reducing the cardiovascular outcomes associated with sleep apnea and improving blood pressure. Stay tuned—more on this in coming years.

40. I read an article about a breathing machine that lowers blood pressure without medication. Should I get one of these devices?

The Resp-e-Rate device is based on a very plausible underlying principle. Recall that the parasympathetic nervous system balances the effects of the sympathetic nervous system. Currently, few drugs effectively leverage the cardiovascular benefits of activating the parasympathetic nervous system. One way in which a person can manipulate both the parasympathetic nervous system and the sympathetic nervous system is by controlled breathing. The Resp-e-Rate machine trains you through musical tones to breathe in a way that tends to reduce the activity of the sympathetic nervous system and stimulate the parasympathetic nervous system, lowering your blood pressure in the process.

A few of my patients have used this device. In some cases, it has helped by virtue of lowering their blood pressure without the need for adding another medicine, which was what I had planned to do until we discussed this option and agreed to it. My only reticence about this device, and other devices likely to appear in the future using this kind of technology, is that we know what kind of benefit blood pressure medications have in terms of reducing heart disease and stroke in hypertension. We do not know whether the same outcomes are likely to occur when blood pressure is lowered by a nondrug mechanism such as one of these machines. On the one hand, the benefit may be the same as—or even better than—that achieved with blood pressure medicines. On the other hand, we may eventually find that these devices are not as good as traditional medications when it comes to long-term outcomes.

Electrocardiogram (EKG or ECG)

A test of the electrical activity of the heart. Little sticky pads are placed at different places on the chest and the electrical activity of the heart is recorded on a piece of special paper. It is also known as an 'EKG' or an 'ECG'. It is used to diagnose things like heart attack and heart wall thickening.

Until more is known about these devices' long-term effectiveness, my recommendation is to cautiously monitor patients with home blood pressure readings who use the Resp-e-Rate. In addition, I recommend keeping tabs on their target organs via traditional tests such as the **electrocardiogram (EKG or ECG)** and blood tests that monitor kidney function to be sure that these functions are not getting worse while we await further studies.

41. Does acupuncture lower blood pressure?

Although some people claim that acupuncture benefits blood pressure, the existing evidence says otherwise. To date, no one has shown a sustained reduction in blood pressure with acupuncture.

PART THREE

Dietary Issues

I feel so relaxed after a few glasses of wine. Does alcohol lower blood pressure?

Can I use special teas, garlic, vitamins, or herbal remedies instead of medications to help my high blood pressure?

Is coffee bad for people with high blood pressure?

More . . .

42. I feel so relaxed after a few glasses of wine. Does alcohol lower blood pressure?

A few years ago I was asked by the Robert Wood Johnson Foundation to review the cardiovascular effects of alcohol, paying particular attention to its impact on blood pressure. What my team found in surveying this area is interesting, and a little paradoxical.

Alcohol actually has two effects on blood pressure. One of these effects was initially hidden from earlier researchers, because they often performed blood pressure measurements 12 to 15 hours after the original alcohol intake. It turns out that this time point coincides with the maximal effect that alcohol has increasing blood pressure. However, when researchers attached a monitor that took study participants' blood pressures multiple times each hour (see Question 11) and measured their blood pressure responses during the time immediately following alcohol ingestion, and *then* continued on to take their blood pressure measurements 12 to 15 hours or more after alcohol intake, a different picture emerged.

Shortly after alcohol ingestion, there is actually a decline in blood pressure. After a few hours, blood pressure returns to its baseline values. As some of the metabolites (the breakdown products of alcohol) then enter into the circulation, there is actually an increase in blood pressure that is evident about 12 to 15 hours after the original alcohol ingestion. Overall, the net effect of alcohol is an increase in blood pressure of about two points, or 2 mm Hg. If you look at the blood pressure 12 to 15 hours after ingestion, this effect appears to be more like 6 mm Hg. Because a 4 mm Hg decrease in blood pressure occurs after ingestion, however, the net increase from alcohol is actually about 2 mm Hg.

How much alcohol is safe to drink? The answer depends on your gender. For men, two or three drinks[1] per day seems to

---

1. A "drink" is one can of beer, one standard mixed drink, or one 6-ounce glass of wine.

be okay. For women, one or two drinks per day is the recommended maximum. These are averages, however. You definitely should *not* have 14 drinks on Saturday and claim that your consumption is an "average of two drinks per day," arguing that the only day you drink is Saturday: The restriction would still be the same even if you drink only one day per week and not all seven. Cut your alcohol consumption off at two or three drinks; your liver and your heart will thank you.

Cut your alcohol consumption off at two or three drinks; your liver and your heart will thank you.

43. Can I use special teas, garlic, vitamins, or herbal remedies instead of medications to help my high blood pressure?

Despite lingering questions about whether dietary supplements actually help with high blood pressure, there's certainly a huge interest in their use. Billions of dollars are spent every year on these so-called nutraceuticals. As with the Resp-e-Rate device mentioned in Question 40, what's missing for these remedies are outcomes studies demonstrating not only the effectiveness of these dietary supplements in reducing blood pressure, but their real benefit in terms of hard outcomes like reduced rates of heart attack and stroke.

In my practice, I do not forbid my patients from taking dietary supplements, but I do insist that "We need to control your blood pressure" and counsel patients to use blood pressure medications in conjunction with any supplements. When patients are able to achieve substantial reductions in blood pressure with these remedies, my first question is whether these decreases are sustained throughout the day or are just transient effects. Home blood pressure measurements can be quite useful in making this determination. Often, these measurements will reveal that these compounds do not lower blood pressure as much as claimed.

In general, these dietary supplements seem have to have very small effects on blood pressure, in the range of 2 to 4 mm Hg. This is about one-half to one-third the reduction in blood

pressure typically achieved with an antihypertensive medication. Also, very few data are available on these remedies'
additive effects—that is, what happens when you use teas
and garlic *and* vitamins *and* other supplements. In addition,
some of these dietary supplements have well-known adverse
effects. In Chinese herb **nephropathy**, for example, Chinese
herbs (which were thought to help general health and blood
pressure) actually damaged the kidney after ingestion because
of a contaminant called aristolochic acid. There have also been
reports of adverse effects from St. John's wort. Clearly, these
supplements are not uniformly benign medications.

If you wish to use dietary supplements in the management
of your blood pressure, you should discuss your plans with
your healthcare provider and agree on a goal. If you're able
to sustain a blood pressure response from these supplements,
you may be fine. Nevertheless, you are taking a risk because
of the long-term benefits (and adverse consequences) of these
compounds remain largely unknown. My advice is to employ
dietary supplements *with*, as opposed to *in place of*, regular
blood pressure medicines.

44. Is coffee bad for people with high blood pressure?

I write this answer while consuming my third cup of coffee
this morning. (That's called a disclaimer.) People who routinely consume regular coffee are relatively unaffected by the
cardiovascular effects of caffeine and all the other stuff in a
cup of coffee. If you're not a regular coffee drinker (I happen
to join the crowd at the espresso bar), you may experience a bit
of a rush from consumption of your brew of choice, complete
with jitters and shakes 20 to 30 minutes after downing that
little bit of brown liquid adulterated to your taste. People who
are not used to caffeine exposure are more likely to experience heart rate increases and blood pressure increases when
they consume caffeine. People who consume caffeine daily, by
contrast, are less likely to see such changes.

Nephropathy

Pertaining to harmful
effects on the kidney.

*If you wish
to use dietary
supplements
in the
management
of your blood
pressure, you
should discuss
your plans with
your healthcare
provider and
agree on a goal.*

Maligning coffee has been the object of medical research for as long as medical research studies have been around. It seems as if every few years or so someone finds a new reason to ding coffee and caffeine. Whether it's linked to hypertension, heart disease, or hangnails, coffee tends to be exonerated in the medical literature within a year or two after an article appears suggesting that it's bad. For those of you who enjoy the brown/black nectar of life (at least for now), salud!

45. My neighbor takes fish oil capsules to reduce her blood pressure. Do they work?

I write an editorial column for the *Journal of Clinical Hypertension*, and have done so pretty much since the journal started in 1999. In my column, I deal with questions and answers related to regular hypertension care. One of the first editorials I wrote addressed this very question. Following are three things that I said in an editorial which I think are still true.

- Fish oil appears to have a small antihypertensive effect when a large dose is used. Achieving this effect may require consumption of 10 capsules daily, which is more than the 1 to 2 capsules commonly recommended. We really don't know exactly how blood pressure is lowered in this case, but fish oil probably behaves similarly to lipid chemicals called **prostaglandins**, which lower blood pressure by acting on specific **receptor** proteins in the blood vessels.
- Studies of the antihypertensive effect of fish oil have mostly examined this supplement's short-term outcome, and there are no long-term outcome studies available. (Did you hear that one before? Revisit Question 43 for the facts on dietary supplements.)
- The use of fish oil is tempered by the unmistakable aromas that exude following the belchings of serious fish oil enthusiasts.

Prostaglandins

These are one of the many lipids in the body.

46. I was told not to eat grapefruit or drink grapefruit juice because of the type of blood pressure medicine I take. Why is that?

Grapefruit juice contains a compound that binds to an enzyme in the liver and intestinal tract. This enzyme, which is called cytochrome p450-3A4 (abbreviated CYP3A4), metabolizes drugs. There's only so much of this enzyme present, so if you saturate it with grapefruit juice and then add certain other medications that also require the enzyme for metabolism, a competition for its attention begins. In this competition, grapefruit juice usually wins. Consequently, drugs that require CYP3A4 for their breakdown accumulate while they wait for an opportunity to be metabolized—an opportunity that comes only after the enzyme system has finished dealing with the grapefruit juice.

The most common types of blood pressure medicines that are affected by grapefruit juice belong to the class called calcium-channel blockers. These drugs include nifedipine, nisoldipine, felodipine, and verapamil, for starters. A listing of these and other grapefruit-sensitive medications is available at online sites such as that operated by the Mayo Clinic (http://www.mayoclinic.com/health/food-and-nutrition/AN00413).

If you take a calcium-channel blocker, you should talk to your about doctor about whether you can safely consume grapefruit juice and take your medication. In the meantime, it's probably a good idea to avoid grapefruit if you take either calcium-channel blockers or statins (cholesterol-lowering medications).

Very commonly, your pharmacist will give you an information sheet that mentions dietary restrictions when you fill your **prescriptions.** Unfortunately, this valuable information is often buried in the fine print. However, some bottles are now labeled with a yellow or pink sticker that warns you when grapefruit consumption should be avoided in conjunction with a particular drug.

It's a good idea to avoid grapefruit if you take either calcium-channel blockers or statins.

Prescription

An instruction from a licensed clinician like a physician, an advanced practice nurse, a midwife, or a physician's assistant that provides for a medication or device to be issued by a pharmacy.

PART FOUR

Medication– Related Issues

How will I know when I need to start taking blood pressure medication, especially if my blood pressure fluctuates?

Will I always have to take medication?

If I miss a dose of my blood pressure medication, should I take twice as much the next time?

More . . .

47. How will I know when I need to start taking blood pressure medication, especially if my blood pressure fluctuates?

This is a tough question, and opinions vary among doctors as to the best answer. My own bias is to begin therapy sooner rather than later, even allowing for the fluctuations. The current threshold at which treatment for high blood pressure begins (140/90 mm Hg) may mean waiting too long in some people, because there will inevitably be a period of time when these individuals' blood pressures will be much higher than the ideal level of less than 115/75 mm Hg. Even when a person's blood pressure falls back into the normal range once in a while, the presence of values in the hypertensive range usually indicates that the person is destined to have high blood pressure someday. If the patient's family history is positive for hypertension (a risk factor for later development of hypertension in the individual), then I am even more strongly inclined to begin therapy early.

If patients are highly motivated and willing to try hard to make lifestyle changes, and their blood pressures are not remarkably elevated, their physicians are often willing to wait months or even up to a year before medications are started.

If patients are highly motivated and willing to try hard to make lifestyle changes, and their blood pressures are not remarkably elevated, their physicians are often willing to wait months or even up to a year to try and maximize the benefit of the lifestyle interventions on blood pressure before medications are started. By contrast, when someone fails to lose weight, appears to be eating as much salt as ever, is not exercising, and so on, the threshold to start medication therapy may be quite low.

Several other factors are usually taken into account when the decision is made to start medication. Often physicians will evaluate an electrocardiogram for signs of blood pressure effects on the heart. These changes might include evidence of heart thickening (hypertrophy) and signs of other heart damage such as silent heart attacks in the past. In addition, blood tests for cholesterol, glucose or sugar, and markers of kidney function may provide data that inform the decision to prescribe medication.

All of these testing procedures are weighed in the balance when it comes to the decision to start a patient on blood pressure medication. The decision-making process is not a pure science, but the physician's goal is always to keep the patient's long-term best interest at the center of the decision. The longer blood pressure therapy is withheld, and the longer the circulation is exposed to abnormally high levels of blood pressure (even if these increases are transient), the more concern grows that the small changes in the blood vessel walls produced by these transient increases in blood pressure will make it more difficult to achieve longer-term blood pressure control with medicines. For that reason, I like to start my patients on medical therapy earlier rather than later. It's akin to the old saying, "An ounce of prevention is worth a pound of cure."

48. Will I always have to take medication?

In most cases, medication must be continued for life. Several medical studies have examined the effects of discontinuing antihypertensive medications and putting patients on rigid regimens designed to maximize the lifestyle approach to blood pressure control. In general, fairly highly motivated people participate in these kinds of studies, but even then the majority of people end up back on blood pressure medicines at some point. Depending on the study, one-half to two-thirds of the participants typically resume drug treatment within four years of trying to get off medication in the first place. Some people do appear to be able to safely withdraw from their medications when they make and adhere to aggressive lifestyle changes, so we can't make a blanket statement about this issue.

In most cases, medication must be continued for life.

When is it safe to withdraw medication? I consider this route when a patient has blood pressures that are repeatedly much lower than expected—for example, 110/70 mm Hg—while taking a single blood pressure medicine. In that situation it's possible the patient could discontinue taking the drug. Once in a great while, someone is misdiagnosed with hypertension. Withdrawal of medication is very likely to work in these individuals, although they don't come in with little signs tattooed on their forehead that say, "I was misdiagnosed with high blood pressure so please stop my medicine." This is—again—why it's so important to correctly diagnose hypertension in the first place by taking multiple readings of a person's blood pressure on multiple occasions.

49. If I miss a dose of my blood pressure medication, should I take twice as much the next time?

What you should do when you miss a dose of your blood pressure medicine depends on *when* you discover you missed the dose. If you realize at 5:00 P.M. that you missed your 8:00 A.M. dose earlier the same day, then taking half the usual amount would make sense. If it's 8:00 A.M. on Wednesday and you just remembered that you forgot to take your medicine on 8:00 A.M. on Tuesday, just take your usual dose on Wednesday and don't double it.

Will it hurt if you take twice the usual dose after forgetting to take your medication on one day? Usually the answer is no, although some blood pressure medicines are more likely to give you trouble if you double the dose in this situation. Perhaps the most important of these medications are drugs like clonidine (Catapres) and labetalol (Normodyne, Trandate). These kinds of drugs tend to have dose-related effects on blood pressure, so you might see your blood pressure drop more than usual if you doubled their doses.

50. If my blood pressure readings are great, can I skip my medicine for a few days?

If you presented to the hospital with pneumonia, and your fever disappeared after 12 hours of penicillin, would you stop the penicillin at that point, even though we know it generally takes seven days' worth of therapy (or more) to truly wipe out the infection? If you're experiencing good blood pressure control and not having side effects from the medications, skipping medications is akin to rocking the boat. The more your blood pressure tolerably approximates normal, the better you will tend to do over the long term, particularly if you have a disorder such as diabetes or kidney disease. If you have symptoms such as dizziness, then your blood pressure regimen may need to be adjusted, but it's not wise to skip your medication altogether.

Some medications may produce rebound blood pressure increases if their use is discontinued abruptly. These drugs include clonidine and some of the beta blockers. If you need to stop taking these medications, your doctor will usually taper them over one to two weeks rather than suddenly interrupting therapy with them.

If you skip your antihypertensive medication, you may find that your blood pressure goes back up and then stays up as you restart your medications. There is a certain amount of lag time between medication administration and achieving and maintaining blood pressure control—which is yet another reason not to interrupt therapy. Like most doctors, I have a handful of patients who are on, well, *unique* regimens crafted to their individual blood pressure profiles. But these regimens are usually developed on a case-by-case basis, in conjunction with home blood pressure monitoring.

51. How do I know if I'm overtreated and taking too much medication?

There are a few signs that you can look for that might indicate your antihypertensive regimen is lowering your blood pressure too much. The most obvious sign is dizziness, which can progress to actually passing out in rare circumstances. These symptoms are more common in elderly patients, particularly after they consume large meals. To fully address this question, we'll develop a checklist.

1. **How low is my blood pressure most of the time?** If your blood pressure is typically less than 100/70 mm Hg, your medication regimen may be a little bit too strong. If you have no symptoms, that would be a judgment call. One group of patients in whom physicians pursue aggressive blood pressure lowering is in persons with diabetes. There are some doctors who would be glad to see a blood pressure in this range, as long as there was no dizziness or passing out, in someone with diabetes.

2. **Have I been lightheaded, particularly when going from lying down to sitting or standing up?** This isn't necessarily a sign of being overtreated. Sometimes dizziness on changing position results from age, diabetes, and disorders that affect the involuntary nervous system (and the activity of the baroreceptor system; see Question 36). It is possible, though, that blood pressure medications may impair some of the reflexes the body uses when changing position and may contribute to lightheadedness, dizziness, or even fainting. These symptoms are more likely to occur following an illness such as a viral infection of the gastrointestinal tract that includes a day or two of nausea and/or diarrhea, which may cause you to become depleted of water and salt and leave you vulnerable to these kinds of symptoms. When you replenish your body's store of salt and water, the symptoms will usually disappear. Their melting away tells you that the culprit is not overtreatment with blood pressure medicines, but rather the intercurrent illness.

3. **Have I passed out or fallen and injured myself?** These events are serious and should definitely lead you to contact your primary care provider. Sometimes they result from blood pressure medicines; at other times they are due to cardiovascular disorders such as severe heart skipping or other issues.

4. **Do I have extreme fatigue in the afternoon to the point where I have to take a nap?** This problem is sometimes due to medications (especially when you take several of them) hitting you all at once. Rather

than reducing or stopping your medications altogether, it is sometimes possible to adjust the timing of the drugs (giving some at night, for example) so as to alleviate such fatigue.

In summary, sometimes patients are genuinely overtreated. Physicians make these determinations on a case-by-case basis. Keep in mind, though, that other factors may also explain what you're experiencing.

52. Do all medications have side effects?

Yes. Every medication, from aspirin to Tylenol (acetaminophen), carries the potential of making someone feel unwell. Blood pressure medicines are relatively potent, because they are meant to make a significant difference in how the heart and blood vessels are working. Because they are so powerful, it makes intuitive sense that they have other effects besides just lowering blood pressure. Moreover, the typical tablet or capsule you take is really a mixture of several components along with the blood pressure medicine; these extras (called excipients) include things like lactose, cellulose and other starches, and minerals. As a result, there's lots of opportunities for you to experience a side effect when you take one of these medicines.

Every medication carries the potential of making someone feel unwell. Nevertheless, most people take blood pressure medicines and feel just fine.

The good news is that most people take blood pressure medicines and feel just fine. Moreover, if you feel unwell on one medication, it's usually possible to substitute or switch to something else and achieve blood pressure benefit with a minimum of impairment in quality of life.

Naturally, a spectrum of adverse effects is associated with the various **classes of blood pressure medications.** Some of the older drugs, for example, were notorious for making people feel poorly. As years have gone by and new medications have been introduced, however, drugs have gotten much more specific for the target system that is blocked so as to lower blood pressure. An example will explain how this works.

Classes of blood pressure medications

There are about eight classes of blood pressure medicines (see Figure 2). ACE-inhibitors block the Angiotensin-Converting Enzyme which reduces the production of angiotensin-II. Angiotensin Receptor Blockers (ARBs) block the binding of angiotensin-II to its receptor (see Receptor) on the blood vessel cell. Alpha1-blockers inhibit adrenaline effects on the blood vessel. Beta-blockers inhibit adrenaline effect on heart muscles. Alpha2-agonists (like clonidine) suppress adrenergic activity. Calcium channel blockers directly relax arterial blood vessels by blocking channels through which calcium enters blood vessels cells. See Diuretics. Vasodilators also directly relax blood vessels cells.

In the past, it was fashionable to use drugs that blocked a significant component of the sympathetic nervous system. These ganglionic blockers were specifically aimed at the little relay stations in the sympathetic nervous system known as ganglia. While they did lower blood pressure, the ganglionic blockers produced a huge number of symptoms because they blocked vital aspects of the sympathetic nervous system other than those affecting the blood pressure. For starters, they caused trouble with the bowels, bladder, vision, and salivation. Moreover, although they did a good job in blocking the ganglia, it was sometimes quite difficult to remain standing up after taking these medications because (as mentioned in Question 20) the sympathetic nervous system is important in adapting our circulation to the upright position.

The most recently introduced class of antihypertensive medications consists of the angiotensin receptor blockers. Of all **classes of blood pressure medications**, they tend to have the least side effects (though they certainly do not completely lack side effects). Naturally, every time someone says something like this, a new class of blood pressure medications is introduced. True to form, a brand-new class of blood pressure medications is due to hit the marketplace shortly. These so-called direct renin inhibitors (DRIs) seem to be similar to the angiotensin receptor blockers in terms of their side-effect profiles, but it's still too early to tell precisely what unwanted symptoms they may produce.

You might wonder why physicians prescribe these medications when we know that a patient might have an adverse reaction to them. This gets at a significant question that's always present in the management of any problem including hypertension—namely, the risk–benefit ratio. The operating principle in this situation is that the benefit we anticipate from treating elevated blood pressure with medications far outweighs the risk of making someone feel poorly in the process.

53. Do I have to keep taking my medications even if I feel bad?

It depends on how bad you feel as to whether you can tough it out until your next opportunity to renegotiate your medication with your prescribing physician. More than 80 blood pressure medications are currently available, so it's usually possible to find something that someone can tolerate and that lowers his or her blood pressure.

Symptoms associated with medication usage tend to come in a couple of flavors. One kind is visible and objective: a rash. That reaction is hard to deny. The rash from drugs is usually a bit like measles, consisting of small, raised red spots. In other circumstances, the symptoms consist of headache, fatigue, or just "not feeling good." These reactions are more subjective, and it's more challenging to sort out what role the blood pressure medicine plays in their occurrence. If you didn't have the symptoms before you took the medicine but the symptoms occur after each dose, that's strong evidence implicating the medicine.

Most of the time, especially if the symptoms are particularly troublesome, the best move is to stop taking the medicine after informing your physician of the problem. Some types of blood pressure medicines really should be tapered rather than suddenly discontinued. Reread the answer to Question 50 just to be on the safe side in case you happen to be taking one of those pills.

The main thing is not to feel imprisoned by your blood pressure medication regimen. Because hypertension tends to stick around for the rest of your life, it's important to work out an equitable arrangement in terms of your medicines that both allows you to function reasonably well and gets the job done controlling your blood pressure.

54. How do I deal with my family and friends when they try to tell me which medications I should be taking?

High blood pressure is so common that many people take antihypertensive medicines. Sometimes it can be quite a challenge to find something that a particular patient can take and that works for him or her. It makes sense that people in your life may want to share their success stories with you to save you from all the headaches that they have been through. But you are not them. While you may appreciate their advice, each person is a unique individual. What works for some doesn't necessarily work for others. My advice is to thank those people for their concern and interest and mumble something like "Gee, I'll have to bring that up with my doctor at the next visit." This way you've acknowledged their concern, but allowed for the option of discussing your medications further with your healthcare provider before any changes are made.

One thing I strongly discourage is striking out on your own when it comes to blood pressure medications. Sometimes medications (blood pressure drugs as well as medications prescribed for other conditions) can interact in such a way that might, for example, slow your heart down too much, to the point where you get extremely tired. Doctors know about these interactions, but well-meaning friends and family don't necessarily have the same kind of pharmacology background. The best advice is to keep an open mind, but make no actual changes in your medications until you have the blessing of your physician.

55. Are generic drugs as good as brand-name drugs?

Yes, according to the U.S. Food and Drug Administration (FDA). This federal agency is charged not only with making sure that drugs are safe, but also with ensuring that generic drugs are equally potent to the brand-name drugs for which they are substituted. The FDA does not require 100% equivalence before it will approve a generic drug, however; the equivalence can range from 80% to 120%. Even so, generic antihypertensive drugs have generally succeeded in maintaining blood pressure control when patients are switched to them from the brand-name compounds. In some cases, the generic drug is actually very similar to the brand-name drug, and sometimes it is actually manufactured by the same company that makes the brand-name medication (although it may be distributed by a different company). In this case, the situation is kind of like buying the store brand, but the product was actually produced by the original maker.

In my practice, some of my patients who switched to the generic drug have occasionally experienced problems that were not present when they took the brand-name medication. This is definitely the exception rather than the rule in my experience. Many patients are actually glad to switch to the generic form because it is usually cheaper.

56. What can I do if I cannot afford my medications?

Several options are available to you when finances are tough and you have trouble paying for your blood pressure medicines. Some doctors have access to drug samples and can supply you for free for at least a little while to see how you do on a particular medication. This practice is, however, becoming less frequent because of all the regulations involved in storing and distributing medication samples.

Some drug companies sponsor programs that provide assistance to patients who have difficulty affording their medications. These programs usually involve a voucher system, and most doctors are aware of companies that provide these services. If you have computer access, you may be able to find which companies offer such benefits by looking at their Web sites.

Other options include visiting a social worker, who may be able to point you in directions that will enable you to get free or lower-priced blood pressure medications. Sometimes you may be eligible to participate in a research study involving blood pressure medication therapies. **Placebo**-controlled trials lasting years are no longer the norm in hypertension research. Instead, modern-day blood pressure medication trials compare one active blood pressure medication regimen against another active blood pressure medication regimen. Such trials may actually go on for several years, and the goal is always to control your blood pressure in these studies, which is typically done at no cost to you for the medications.

Placebo

Usually an inactive substance that contains no medication or active ingredient to be given to participants in a clinical trial to determine the effectiveness of a particular medication or substance.

57. If I need a certain medication, but it causes side effects, what can be done?

Most medications are members of a particular class of drugs. For example, the angiotensin-converting enzyme (ACE) inhibitor class includes approximately 10 drugs. The names of the drugs in this class all end with the letters "pril"—for example, captopril, enalapril, and ramipril. When you need a certain medication but it has side effects, then, your first option (plan A) is to consider using a different agent within the same class. If someone had a side effect of nausea when taking enalapril, for example, he or she might be switched to ramipril or lisinopril.

In some cases, all of the members of a particular drug class produce the same side effect—that is, a class effect. Continuing to use the ACE inhibitor analogy, if someone had a cough on enalapril, the cough would likely return if the patient switched to ramipril, because this side effect tends to happen with all ACE inhibitors.

That brings us to plan B. In plan B, we try to substitute a member of a drug class that is similar in its goals as the parent class with a side effect. As an example, angiotensin receptor blockers are somewhat similar to ACE inhibitors in their mode of action and are considered an acceptable substitute for ACE inhibitors—but they don't usually produce a cough. Thus the second option is to look within a class of medications that are somewhat similar to the class for which a side effect occurred.

Plan C (the third-line option) is to give the drug in divided doses instead of all at once. Sometimes side effects are a result of the amount of medication given, so splitting the dose may allow the drug to be continued with less impairment in someone's well-being. Along these lines, you can sometimes use a side effect to your advantage. If you take a medication first thing in the morning and feel really tired around 9:00 or 10:00 A.M., that sort of medication might be able to be dosed at night; the tiredness you feel would then occur at a time when you're planning to go to sleep anyway.

58. Will blood pressure medication affect my sexual desire or my ability to perform sexually?

Sexual desire and sexual performance are incredibly complicated issues, so this is one of the toughest questions to answer with a simple yes or no. A great deal of attention has been devoted to this topic, and many articles have been written about the effect of blood pressure medications on sexual performance and sexual desire (known as libido). Moreover, it is likely that the way in which a particular drug affects sexual aspects of a person's life differs depending on whether you are a man or a woman.

Sexual function includes both significant psychological aspects and important physical aspects. Some blood pressure medicines do interfere with the involuntary nervous system and could, therefore, impair the responses and changes needed to engage in sex. Other medications—diuretics, for example—do not interfere with the physical mechanisms needed to prepare for sex, but nonetheless are associated with a small but definite rate of difficulty in achieving an erection.

Some year ago I was part of a research team that conducted the Treatment of Mild Hypertension Study (TOMHS). In this study, people aged 45 or older with hypertension were treated with either a sugar pill and lifestyle changes (see Question 23) or one of five different blood pressure medication classes and lifestyle changes; the goal was to see how much added benefit the drugs would provide over the lifestyle changes alone. One of the things we did was to assess the effect of therapy on sexual performance by using a blinded design—that is, neither the doctors nor the patients knew what any one person in the study was getting (we knew only that any one person had a definite chance of being on placebo or being on one or the other of the active medications). The TOMHS investigation tested a placebo (a sugar pill) against a diuretic (chlorthalidone), a beta blocker (acebutalol), an alpha blocker (doxazosin), an ACE inhibitor (enalapril), and a calcium-channel blocker (amlodipine). Here's what we found (this is from the abstract of the published study, which appeared in the journal *Hypertension* in 1997; http://www.ncbi.nlm.nih.gov/entrez/query.fcgi?db=pubmed&cmd=Retrieve&dopt=AbstractPlus&list_uids=9039073&query_hl=13&itool=pubmed_docsum):

In many cases, erection dysfunction did not require withdrawal of medication. Disappearance of erection problems among men with problems at baseline was common in all groups but greatest in the doxazosin group. Incidence of reported sexual problems in women was low in all treatment groups. In conclusion, long-term incidence of erection problems in treated hypertensive men is relatively low but is higher with chlorthalidone treatment. Effects of erection dysfunction with chlorthalidone appear relatively early and are often tolerable, and new occurrences after 2 years are unlikely. The rate of reported sexual problems in hypertensive women is low and does not appear to differ by type of drug. Similar incidence rates of erection dysfunction in placebo and most active drug groups caution against routine attribution of erection problems to antihypertensive medication.

59. I don't like swallowing pills. What can I do to get my medication down?

High blood pressure medication comes in a variety of shapes and sizes. There are tablets, capsules, fizzy tablets that dissolve in the fluid of your choice (these are usually potassium supplements), and liquid preparations (mostly for children, alas). Most blood pressure medicines come in pill or capsule form, however.

The first consideration is whether something is wrong with your **esophagus.** Once in a while people develop a stricture, or a narrowing, in their esophagus, usually as the result of years of **acid reflux.** In this situation, deal with the stricture first. This will be the exception rather than the rule, however.

Some patients have dreamed up ingenious ways to get blood pressure medications from their mouth to their stomach. Some crush the pills and hide them in applesauce, for example. One of my patients "buttered" her pills. Some tablets come with a little score down the center so that they can be broken in half. Many blood pressure medicines can simply be crushed and mixed with a fruit drink or plain water and swallowed it that way.

But be aware that there are several medications with which this approach should not be tried. These exceptions arise because of the way the tablet is made. Several blood pressure medicines use a timed-release tablet formulation; it is not advisable to break or crush these kinds of medications. Usually your pharmacist can tell you whether your blood pressure medicine falls into this category.

An example is the pill called nifedipine-GITS (brand name: Procardia GITS). (Here "GITS" is not a derogatory term referring to a group of fools in a Monty Python skit but rather an acronym referring to gastrointestinal therapeutic system.)

Esophagus

The swallowing tube or passageway that connects the mouth with the stomach.

Acid reflux

When the sphincter which separates the stomach from the esophagus is lax, stomach acid leads backward, or 'refluxes' up the esophagus. This acid reflux causes heartburn and sometimes a narrowing or stricture in the esophagus that can interfere with swallowing.

The goal in such preparations is to take a drug that is relatively short acting but to capitalize on a sustained release that slows delivery of the active ingredient in an effort to prolong its effect on blood pressure.

One of the downsides to opening a capsule, dropping its contents into a fluid, and then swallowing it, or doing essentially the same thing to a tablet by virtue of dissolving it in a liquid, is that the resulting drink may have an unpleasant "medicine" taste. In this case, no matter how hard you squeeze your nose and swallow, there may be some aftertaste issues. Even so, it may still be worth a try when the type of tablet or capsule formulation allows such handling, provided your friendly neighborhood pharmacist doesn't expressly say otherwise.

60. If I have to take medications for other conditions such as arthritis, diabetes, or heart disease, can I take all of my pills at the same time?

Fortunately, most blood pressure medicines nowadays don't have a characteristic peak effect. When a drug is being studied for high blood pressure, one of the things the FDA evaluates is the amount of blood pressure reduction at both the peak (the greatest effect) and the trough (the end of the proposed dosing cycle). The goal of such an evaluation is to make sure that the blood pressure reduction at the end of the dosing interval (for example, at 8:00 A.M. following a dose yesterday at 8:00 A.M. when the proposed dosing interval is once a day) is not due to an excessively large effect at the peak blood pressure time (which is often about eight hours after the dose is taken) in products seeking a once-daily indication. Most antihypertensive drugs available today have fairly equivalent peak and trough effects, so they rarely interfere with other drugs when it comes to symptoms.

There are important considerations related to drug interactions with antihypertensive medications, however. That is, other medicines that you take for other conditions may affect your blood pressure. You might recall the withdrawal of Vioxx (rofecoxib) from the marketplace several years ago.

Vioxx was prescribed to patients with arthritis as a pain reliever, but it also increased blood pressure. For similar reasons, physicians carefully monitor their patients who take multiple medications given the possibility of a drug interaction where treatment for other conditions may affect blood pressure.

Of course, drug interactions cut both ways. Sometimes blood pressure medicines may influence the blood sugar concentration, so diabetes medicines may need to be adjusted in some circumstances. Also, sometimes blood pressure medicines work in a "two for" fashion—for example, they may treat not only hypertension but also heart failure or coronary artery disease.

You should read all of those little decals plastered on your medication bottle, because occasionally the label will say something like "take this [pill or capsule] at" certain times, such as before or after a meal or other medications. The other place to look for information is in the patient package insert; your pharmacist may staple it to the bag containing your medication. You might need a magnifying glass to read the small print, but the section on drug interactions might provide valuable information.

61. My doctor says I need additional medication to control my blood pressure. Why not just increase the dose of the single medicine I'm on now?

There are two reasons why it's usually a better move to add another medication, rather than to titrate the existing drug to its maximum dosage when you're taking a single blood pressure medicine.

The first reason is that most of the blood pressure benefit (80% to 90%) is achieved when you take approximately half the maximal dose. Consequently, increasing the dose to maximum (or beyond) usually results in an additional reduction in blood pressure of only 2 to 3 mm Hg.

The second reason has to do with adverse effects—the things that make patients feel bad. These potential problems are usually listed in long columns in the patient package insert (see Question 60). As a rule, many (though not all) adverse effects are dose-related. If the dose of the medication is increased to the maximum, you may achieve a few more points in blood pressure reduction but often at the risk of feeling less well because of the adverse effects.

In most cases, adding a second blood pressure medicine to a patient's drug regimen leads to a much greater reduction in blood pressure than increasing the dose of the first medicine.

In most cases, adding a second blood pressure medicine to a patient's drug regimen leads to a much greater reduction in blood pressure than increasing the dose of the first medicine. Many blood pressure medicines are now available in what are called a combination formulation. When you find out how well you do on a second medication, the first medication you were given might be available with the second medication built into it, so you have to take only one pill rather than two.

62. Do some medications increase blood pressure?

Let's split this answer into two parts. The first part will assume that we're talking about a blood pressure medicine. The second part will cover some of the common drugs that increase blood pressure as a side effect.

Most blood pressure medications do what they are supposed to do: lower blood pressure. If you read the package insert carefully, however, you may sometimes see a phrase such as "increases in blood pressure" listed in the adverse effects section. Why? Blood pressure is subject to variability (see Question 8). Sometimes blood pressure may actually be higher—not lower—after medications are started. For one class of blood pressure medicines, this effect occurs a bit more often than blood pressure variability would explain—namely, when beta blockers are given to African American patients. Not only do these drugs not lower blood pressure in some patients, but occasionally patients' blood pressure might actually increase after they take beta blockers. This relationship has been found in several clinical trials, so it doesn't appear to be a fluke. Fortunately, it's relatively uncommon, occurring in fewer than 5% of people. Given this possibility, most doctors would not prescribe a beta blocker as first-line antihypertensive therapy in an African American patient unless there were other reasons to use this medication, such as to prevent migraine headache or treat heart disease.

Increases in blood pressure can occur with several commonly used types of medications. Arthritis medicines can have this effect, for example, as can most medications other than aspirin or Tylenol (acetaminophen) that are used to treat chronic pain. This effect can usually be eliminated by adjusting the blood pressure medicines when it's not possible to stop the pain relievers. Other examples of medications that can increase blood pressure include cough-cold preparations that contain decongestant medications. If you buy these over-the-counter medications, try to purchase the short-acting versions rather than the long-acting kinds. In my practice, I try not to use these medications at all, but once in a while I give in when someone is truly miserable.

The following list highlights some other occasions when medicines might raise blood pressure:

- Some anticancer agents (for example, Avastin or Prednisone)
- Drugs used to prevent organ transplant rejection (for example, cyclosporine or tacrolimus)
- Drugs used to treat migraine headaches (for example, Imitrex)

This doesn't mean you can *never* use these medicines if you have high blood pressure. The choice of a medication that might increase blood pressure depends on the risk–benefit trade-off. Sometimes physicians prescribe medications with known side effects when the good the drugs will do outweighs their risks to the patient.

63. If I am an African American patient, should I be on different medications than a white, Hispanic American, or Asian American patient?

When a patient with hypertension is taking a single medication to control his or her blood pressure, studies show that some types of medicines work better in certain ethnic groups compared to other ethnic groups. For example, diuretics tend to work better in African American patients than in white patients, at least when the patients are younger than 60 years of age. Conversely, ACE inhibitors tend to be more effective in white or Asian American patients compared to African American patients. Of course, some African American patients may respond well to ACE inhibitors and less well to diuretics. The trends identified here are based on percentages in the medical research literature: While they may hold true in the aggregate, there is always room for an individual choice when it comes to managing each person's blood pressure.

When physicians add a second pressure medicine to an established first-line medicine, most of the ethnic differences in blood pressure response to medications usually go away. Their disappearance has to do with the two drugs' ability to leverage complementary means by which a blood pressure is reduced. Recall that effective high blood pressure management relies on medications that treat different blood pressure servos (see Figure 2 in Question 14). Thus using drugs with different mechanisms of action is much more likely to get the blood pressure down than piling on medications that work on the same side of that four-sided figure.

Research shows that different servos play different roles in the development of hypertension in some ethnic groups compared to others. For example, African American patients are more likely to be salt-sensitive (see Question 23), so diuretics that reduce the effects of salt on blood pressure have a higher likelihood of working in this ethnic group. White patients, especially when younger, often have high levels of activity in the renin–angiotensin axis, so ACE inhibitors and angiotensin-receptor blockers are statistically more likely to work in these patients as compared to diuretics.

Once you take the plunge and start a medication, the other servos wake up and begin to exert more effort in an effort to pull your blood pressure back up. For example, when an African American patient takes a diuretic, his or her renin–angiotensin axis becomes more active. This phenomenon sets the stage for additional blood pressure reduction with ACE inhibitors, for instance.

64. I am overweight and don't have any luck with diets. My doctor told me that taking diet pills is not a good idea for people with high blood pressure. What's wrong with diet pills?

Question 23 addressed this issue as well. The answer here will expand on this point because it is a common question, and a common concern. You might recall that a few years ago a drug called fenfluramine (Redux) was pulled from the market. The main issue with drug was that its risk–benefit equation no longer seem to favor benefit over risk. This is one of the more common reasons why a drug may be withdrawn from the market. Often it takes several years of clinical usage before drugs' side-effect profiles become fully known. In the case of Redux, concerns arose about the effect it had on blood pressure (in the lung circulation, which is somewhat different than the type of blood pressure covered in this book).

Several types of drugs to reduce weight are available. One group works by imitating chemicals used by the sympathetic nervous system. Using this mechanism of action can raise blood pressure, because that's part of what the sympathetic nervous system does. It is also what amphetamines do, and what Redux did in the lung circulation. You might wonder whether the blood-pressure-raising effects might be balanced by the weight loss associated with these drugs' use. Sometimes they are, but in general the pressure increase gets more of healthcare practitioners' attention when it comes to keeping the best interest of the patient in mind.

Other weight-loss drugs rely on different mechanisms of action. For example, orlistat (Xenical) works by blocking fat absorption in the intestine. These medications also have a small blood-pressure-reducing effect when they successfully produce some weight loss. Their major problems relate to large bowel complaints. Moreover, as mentioned in Question 25, the weight loss induced through use of these drugs is not permanent, because the person's underlying behavior patterns have not changed. Once you lose weight but stop the medication, there's no permanent change in your metabolism—so there's no reason to think the weight will stay off.

The practice of weight cycling—in which patients lose weight, gain it back, lose weight again, and gain it back again—has also created some concerns. Some medical research suggests that this fluctuation in weight may be worse than simply having the weight in the first place. There is no lack of interest in the pharmaceutical industry in finding ways to safely lower weight, improve blood pressure, improve blood sugar and lipid levels, and all the rest with the medication. At this time, the promise of delivering on this indication remains mostly just that—a promise and not a reality.

Virginia comments:

I am unwilling to take additional medication that may cause harm by stimulating the sympathetic nervous system when I really need to work on behavioral issues so that I can both lose the weight and then keep it off. But I am also waiting patiently for the perfect, safe pill that will just do it for me!

65. At what age am I "too old" to need blood pressure medication?

Most of the research studies demonstrating the value of treating high blood pressure cut off the age of entry into the studies to 70 or 75 years. Given that many blood pressure studies are 4 to 5 years long, good information is therefore available on the value of treating high blood pressure up to the age of 80 years or so. Beyond that point, it's largely speculation; there's very little hard evidence about blood pressure management in this crowd.

One thing that many patients with hypertension fear, particularly when they are in this older age range, is that they will have a debilitating stroke but *not* die—that is, that they might end up debilitated and dependent. Medical research shows that older patients are willing to sacrifice years of life to avoid this tragic situation.

A study called the Hypertension in the Very Elderly Trial (HYVET) is now under way to investigate the benefits of treating hypertension in the age 80 and older population. The pilot information for this trial, which the scientists considered while deciding on the feasibility of doing the HYVET study, came to two interesting conclusions. Although these are preliminary findings (that's why the bigger trial is now being done), they are nevertheless quite interesting:

- People older than age 80 who were treated with blood pressure medications tended to die a little earlier compared with those who had hypertension and were not treated.
- People older than age 80 who were treated with blood pressure medications tended to have fewer strokes compared with those who had hypertension and were not treated.

Please keep in mind that these findings are considered suggestive rather than definitive. If you would like to read more about this particular topic, the abstract for this study is cited in the "Literature and Other Sources of Information" appendix at the end of the book.

66. Should I take my blood pressure medicine in the morning or in the evening?

Traditionally, blood pressure medication has been dosed in the morning.

Traditionally, blood pressure medication has been dosed in the morning. Indeed, most clinical trials of blood pressure therapies have used this kind of regimen. Of course, there is always room for improvement on a case-by-case basis, so let's look at a few examples.

Some medications tend to have some tiredness or fatigue associated with their use. These kinds of medicines, if used in a once-daily fashion, could be given at night, in which case this potential adverse effect might work to your advantage and help you sleep.

Some limited medical research suggests that some patients experience a substantial rise in their blood pressure after getting up in the morning, compared to their blood pressure shortly before getting out of bed. You may not know your blood pressure while you are sleeping, but you can check it about the time you are due to take your next daily blood pressure medication dose. If your pressures are higher than 140/90 mm Hg on most mornings but look fine in the afternoon and evening, it may help either to take your medicine in the evening or to split the dose and take half in the morning and half in the evening.

One interesting question in the care of patients with hypertension relates to the finding—of which most people are aware—that most heart attacks occur between getting up in the morning and noon. What we are lacking in hypertension care is good evidence that specifically targeting this time period, with the antihypertensive drug being taken at nighttime as opposed to in the morning, will reduce this well-known healthcare statistic. At the present time, we are just not sure whether changing the timing of the medications will alter this trend. Consequently, we tend to adjust medications and use an evening dose mostly to treat side effects or to counteract high blood pressures in the morning. That may change as the results of new clinical studies are published. Stay tuned.

67. If I feel bad, how do I know whether it's a side effect of my blood pressure medicine?

Some types of blood pressure medications have well-known side-effect profiles. For example, use of the angiotensin-converting enzyme (ACE) inhibitors is associated with an annoying cough. Another common side effect is swelling of the feet as the day goes on, a phenomenon that is seen with calcium-channel blockers. **Table 1** indicates the more common side effects that are seen with the major blood pressure medication classes.

Table 1

Drug class	Example	Side effect	Frequency*
Diuretic	HCTZ, Hydrodiuril ®	Low potassium	5%
Beta-blocker	Inderal ®	Fatigue	5%
Alpha-blocker	Cardura ®	Dizziness	1-4%
ACE-inhibitor	Capoten ®, Altace ®	Cough	7-9%
Calcium	Isopten ® (verapamil)	Constipation	10%
Channel	Cardizem ® (diltiazem)		
Blockers	Procardia ®, Norvasc ®	Ankle Swelling	5-10%
Angiotensin Receptor Blockers	Cozaar ®, Diovan ®	Dizziness	1-2%
Alpha-2 Agonists	Catapres ®	Dry mouth	5-10%
Vasodilators	Loniten ®	Swelling	> 10%

*Frequency is dependent on age and doses used

Some people experience other side effects that don't appear in Table 1. These come in several varieties. Some side effects are what we call objective (that is, observable)—for example, a rash. Other side effects are subjective—for example, nausea. This side effect may occur either because the person's stomach is completely empty or because he or she really does get a nauseated feeling when taking blood pressure (or other) medications.

How do we tell whether the antihypertensive medication is to blame for these side effects? In my practice, I use a four-step process to sort this problem out:

1. Taper (Question 50) and/or stop the medicine and wait a few days to a few weeks.
2. Did the side effect go away?
    (a) Yes: Go to number 3.
    (b) No: Stop here; it may not be the drug.
3. Restart the medication (if this is considered safe to do, in that the side effect was not a life-threatening one).
4. Did the side effect come back?
    (a) Yes: The medication is probably the culprit.
    (b) No: The fault might not lie with the medication (or you may just be lucky and got better).

This is not a foolproof system, of course. One problem that healthcare providers often face in hypertension care is that a patient doesn't take just one medicine, but rather takes many different medications. Consequently, to ferret out whether one or the other of the medications is the culprit, providers make an educated guess as to which one is most likely responsible for the side effect and then put that drug through the four-step sequence outlined above when it is felt safe to do so. Given that one of the biggest issues providers face in hypertension care is getting people to stay committed to their blood pressure medications for the long term, healthcare providers usually try very hard to deal with side-effect issues and pinpoint the responsible drug, switching to something else whenever possible.

68. Do some blood pressure medications make people gain weight?

Most blood pressure medications are weight-neutral. Diuretics are sometimes associated with a small drop in body weight. Conversely, beta blockers are statistically associated with a small weight gain (usually less than 4 to 5 pounds). Most blood pressure medicines will *not* cause a weight gain of 10 or 20 (or more) pounds.

Beta blockers are thought to increase weight in two ways:

- *Decreased metabolism.* When the body's metabolism slows, fewer calories are expended each day. If the person does not change his or her intake, the unused calories will gradually be stored, resulting in the 4- to 5-pound weight gain mentioned previously. Eventually the body strikes a new balance and weight gain stops.
- *Mechanism of action.* The way in which beta blockers work may lead to weight gain. These drugs reduce heart rate most of the time, and they reduce the cardiac output. As a result, the activity level of people often decreases, which may lead to less calorie expenditure and, in turn, increased weight.

With chronic therapy (that is, after the first couple of months), these effects usually go away and further weight increase is usually not seen.

69. My ankles are swollen but the doctor told me not to worry about it because "It's common in people who take that kind of medication." Should I worry anyway?

If you look back at Table 1 (in Question 67), you'll see that one of the side effects associated with calcium-channel blockers is ankle swelling. This kind of ankle swelling usually gets worse during the day, but is much less noticeable in the morning when a person first gets out of bed. It's not usually associated with a weight gain. This kind of swelling can be annoying, but it is rarely a health hazard.

Three kinds of calcium-channel blockers are used to treat high blood pressure. Two of the three kinds— verapamil and diltiazem—have only one chemical agent in their classification; both are available as generic drugs as well. The remaining calcium-channel blockers are more often associated with ankle swelling; they include nifedipine, felodipine, nisoldipine, amlodipine, isradipine, and nicadipine. (Ankle swelling can happen with verapamil and diltiazem, but it isn't as frequently seen with these drugs.)

The swelling associated with these types of calcium-channel blockers is thought to occur because of the distribution of the proteins in the cells of the blood vessels that the calcium-channel blockers "block." Arteries and veins differ in this respect, such that calcium-channel blockers tend to be better at dilating arteries than veins. As a result, when you sit up or stand up, blood will find its way into your legs a little more easily if you are taking a calcium-channel blocker, but the rate at which the blood exits the legs through the veins remains unchanged. The difference in these rates means that a little bit of blood is left behind in the legs because of the relative changes in artery and vein pressures, which in turn results in swelling of the ankles. Once the swelling reaches a certain balance point in any individual during the course of the day, it tends not to get any worse because the lymphatic system kicks into action to prevent further fluid collection.

When you are lying down, gravity is no longer an issue in terms of blood flow. Thus, when you sleep at night, the fluid that built up during the day is usually reabsorbed or distributed to some other place in the body. Sometimes you may notice a need to void urine during the night as you reabsorb those little reservoirs of fluid around your ankles. As far as we know, there are no other consequences of ankle swelling caused by use of calcium-channel blockers aside from the inconvenience of occasionally voiding urine during the night.

Other causes of swelling are possible, however. When the heart, liver, or kidneys have impaired function, for example, their poor performance may result in swelling. Also, pulmonary hypertension—a type of hypertension in which the pressure is abnormally high in the lung circulation—can lead to swelling of the ankles. These conditions are much different and far more serious situations than the ankle swelling linked to typical hypertension medicines. Typically, impaired organ function leaves a trail of clues, such as breathlessness, failure of swelling to improve in the morning, skin yellowing, extreme tiredness, or waking up short of breath in the night. These symptoms are not usually present when swelling is simply a side effect of calcium-channel blocker use. If present, they may be indicators of other, more serious issues deserving further evaluation.

70. I read an article that stated some blood pressure medicines cause diabetes. Is that true?

At least two classes of blood pressure medications have been implicated in raising blood sugar levels: diuretics and beta blockers. Medical researchers are divided in their opinions as to how important drug-induced diabetes (compared to the kind that is not related to high blood pressure medicines) is with respect to important outcomes such as heart disease, stroke, and kidney failure.

When a group of patients with hypertension is followed for 5 to 10 years, quite a few will develop diabetes. As mentioned in Question 24, diabetes is approximately twice as likely to occur when hypertension is already present. Comparisons of different blood pressure medicines in clinical trials of hypertension treatment have also shown that the incidence of diabetes is higher when patients take diuretics or beta blockers compared to other classes of drugs. So where does the debate come in?

At least two classes of blood pressure medications have been implicated in raising blood sugar levels: diuretics and beta blockers.

The debate arises because medical researchers are unsure how ominous developing diabetes as a result of, or in conjunction with, diuretic treatment is with respect to cardiovascular outcomes such as heart attack and stroke. Some research says it has no appreciable effect; other research suggests that there *might* be a link between diuretic-induced diabetes and poorer heart-related outcomes. Only in the last few years has this issue taken center stage in hypertension treatment, and the debate remains to be settled. The question is not so much whether diabetes occurs in conjunction with these antihypertensive medications, but whether the improvement in blood pressure associated with drugs such as diuretics outweighs these drugs' effects on blood sugar levels. At this point, there is more information to support the benefit from the use of diuretics in treating hypertension than there is evidence suggesting that these drugs should be avoided. For now, we still use diuretics routinely in hypertension care.

When it comes to beta blockers, the jury is still out. At least one commonly used beta blocker, atenolol, has not done as well as other therapies in terms of cardiovascular outcomes despite its ability to lower the blood pressure to an equivalent degree as these other agents. By and large, physicians have been moving away from using atenolol as first-line therapy for treating hypertension. At the same, there are solid reasons to continue using atenolol in some people, particularly those with coronary heart disease, faster heart rates, migraine headaches, and several other indications.

71. What should I do when I hear a news story that says my medication causes heart attacks or some other health problem?

About every six months to a year, this kind of thing tends to happen—and it isn't limited to cardiovascular disease, either. Concerns about cancer and other chronic illnesses that none of us wish to have also crop up in the news periodically. Sometimes the news report is quite dramatic and has a huge scare factor associated with it. So how do you deal with the fear it brings?

When I was an intern in Internal Medicine, I read a book called *The House of God* by Samuel Shem. I don't recommend this book for those with a weak constitution because it takes great delight in poking holes in people's concepts of health care in a hospital (in the 1970s). However, one "rule" from *The House of God* is very appropriate to this question: "In a cardiac arrest, take your own pulse first." The application of this bit of wisdom to the current question is this: Ask yourself, "Was I okay five minutes before I heard this broadcast?" If the answer is yes, take a few deep breaths and relax. Odds are you will live safely long enough to discuss this news story with your doctor.

Why do these things happen, anyway? The process by which drugs are approved is one factor. For high blood pressure medications, the approval process is mainly oriented toward demonstrating that the new medication safely and effectively lowers blood pressure. Typically, the drug has been studied in several thousand people, so that its developer has a good idea how well it works, and in whom, and what the common side effects are expected to be. Once in a while, however, unforeseen problems arise when use of the drug is expanded to a much larger population after its approval by the FDA, and these lead to the unfortunate news broadcasts like those that frame this question. Sometimes the news report is verified in other research studies and we believe the findings to be true; in such cases, we make the best choices possible about treatment on a patient-by-patient basis. Sometimes the news report is a bit sensational, and when cooler heads prevail we find that it's mostly much ado about very little.

How can you know whether what you hear applies specifically to you? The short answer is "You probably can't." Many times the findings in these studies apply to relatively small but important subgroups of patients treated with medications. Because so many blood pressure medicines are available, it will usually be possible to switch from one drug to another if your doctor believes in the accuracy of the news story.

My basic advice in this situation is *don't panic*. Also, keep in mind that you probably are not the only person taking this medication as you place that call to your doctor to find out the real story. While you wait for your return phone call, my advice is to have a cup of cocoa: I just finished reviewing an article saying that cocoa lowers blood pressure (in the April 2007 issue of *Archives of Internal Medicine*). This way (as long as you like dark chocolate) you'll be helping your blood pressure, enjoying a scrumptious drink, and doing your best to be calm and relax while you wait for a chance to discuss the latest CNN story with someone from your doctor's office.

72. Why does my pharmacist always give me a list of bad things that drugs do to people?

Patients often bring me these package inserts, which they have usually highlighted with yellow marker followed by several red or black exclamation points. A particular favorite is "death." Fortunately, death is not that common as a side effect of antihypertensive medications, but it certainly does get one's attention.

The pharmacist provides this information in part because it's a component of his or her job. A pharmacist's job is to safely dispense medication, and part of that process means keeping the consumer informed about potential drug interactions, side effects, and important instructions for taking the particular medication. This information may vary from one type of medicine to another.

Keep in mind that when it comes to some of the older blood pressure medicines, such as the diuretics, literally tens of millions of people have been treated with these compounds. It stands to reason that some unusual side effects might have cropped up given all that "opportunity." The FDA and several other regulatory agencies keep a watch over the things that happen to people when they take drugs that have been launched into the marketplace, whether antihypertensive or any other kind of medicine. An elaborate system for reporting side effects has been established, and it is the responsibility of every drug company to take every report seriously—which they usually do. The vast amount of data gathered this way is distilled into the package insert that is stapled to the bag in which the medication bottle is contained when you pick it up at the pharmacy. Some people never read these informational sheets; others people obsess about them.

My advice is to take your medicine as prescribed. If you feel something odd, such as a pain in your side or an itchy section of skin, consider that the cause might be all that snow you shoveled this morning or the poison ivy you pulled up yesterday, as well as your medication that might be causing the side effect. In short, keep things in perspective. After all, it is unlikely that every symptom you will ever experience will be linked to your blood pressure medicine.

I recommend that you keep a package insert for each medication you take. If something does happen and you wonder if it's drug-related, take a look at the sheet and see if the symptom appears there. Next, ask yourself how long you've been taking this medication before the symptom arose. If you've been taking the medicine for years, it's less likely that the drug is responsible for the new symptom. If you're relatively new to the medication and your symptom appears on the package insert list (and particularly when it affected more than 5% of patients in the clinical trials), perhaps the medication is to blame. Your healthcare providers' goal is to manage your blood pressure both as comfortably and as effectively as possible, so they will take side effects seriously, and try to make changes when possible.

It is unlikely that every symptom you will ever experience will be linked to your blood pressure medicine, so the best advice is to take your medicine as prescribed.

Medication-Related Issues

73. My insurance company no longer pays for the medication my doctor has prescribed for me in the past and has recommended an alternative. Should I switch to it?

Most of the time, it's perfectly reasonable to make the change. It is irritating when those changes are made every year or two as the winds of insurance agencies change based upon the prevailing cost benefits they are able to negotiate with drug suppliers. Within most classes of antihypertensive medications, all of the agents with the same class typically achieve relatively similar degrees of blood pressure lowering.

There is one reason to keep someone on a particular type of blood pressure medicine even if it is not covered by his or her insurer. Some medications have really been put to the acid test with respect to their use in specific circumstances—for example, in clinical research studies of diabetes and hypertension with the outcome being changes in kidney function over time. Such studies are expensive, so these expensive studies were clearly undertaken to answer a clinically important question. It may be that any other agent in the same class might produce the same outcome. Until the research studies are done, however, you don't know that; you can only assume it is true because the drug is a member of the same class.

When I believe a particular drug is important for a specific aspect of a patient's high blood pressure care, I will try to persuade the insurer to make an exemption and support the use of a brand-name product that is not currently on the insurer's list of approved medications (called a **formulary**). In my practice, this probably happens 5% to 10% of the time when the insurer mandates a switch. Like most doctors, my inbox for snail mail overflows with notes from various insurers about what's on their formularies and what I've prescribed for individual patients. Insurance companies cannot be blamed for trying to make these changes. After all, they are trying to run their businesses in the most fiscally responsible manner

Formulary

A listing of drugs or medications available for dispensing by either a pharmacy, a hospital or a prescription warehouse.

possible. Although their orders may be irritating, most of the time (as long as the patient is agreeable) I'll go along with the switch unless I have a strong feeling otherwise.

Sometimes the switch doesn't work out: The patient either doesn't do as well on the new drug or he or she experiences a side effect that didn't occur with the original medication. This outcome usually makes it easier to get an exemption, but paperwork and often some time on hold on the phone are usually needed to accomplish it.

74. My lower blood pressure number is fine, but my doctor says that at my age the upper number is more important and we need to get that down, too. Isn't a lower number less than 90 mm Hg pretty good?

For many years, physicians considered the lower blood pressure number (the **diastolic** value) to be far more important than the upper number (the **systolic** value). This kind of thinking came into vogue in the first half of the twentieth century and persisted until the 1990s, when the results of a study called the Systolic Hypertension in the Elderly Program (SHEP) were published. This study was responsible for changing medical thinking on two fronts:

- It provided evidence, for the first time, that treating an elevated upper number when the lower number was normal reduced heart attack and stroke, and significantly so.
- It showed that it was, indeed, safe to treat older people (in whom elevated upper numbers and normal to low numbers are more common).

In the latter case, the word "safe" means two things. First, there appears to be no adverse consequence to treating an older person with blood pressure medication in terms of outcomes: The stroke, heart attack, and heart failure rates were all lower

Diastolic

The period of time when the heart is not actively contracting. In a blood pressure value like 134/76 mm Hg the "76" is the diastolic value (the 134 is the systolic value).

Systolic

The period when the heart is actively contracting. With a blood pressure like 126/88 mm Hg the 126 represents the systolic value (the 88 is the diastolic value).

when patients in the SHEP study received active medication treatment as compared with a placebo. Second, patients in the SHEP study did not have frequent falls and hip fractures. Prior to the publication of the SHEP study, this possibility had been cited as a reason to avoid treating older patients with high blood pressure where the upper number is the problem and the lower number is normal.

Blood pressure numbers go up for two main reasons. When you're relatively young (for example, less than 50 years old), the lower number is remarkably important for predicting heart attack and other problems associated with high blood pressure. Recall the answer to Question 2, which noted that the lower number reflects the "spigot" aspect of the circulation. When the lower number is high, it's more difficult to force fluid—in this case, blood—through the system. The additional work puts a strain on the heart and the circulation, and leads to the attendant problems of heart attack, heart failure, and so on. When people are relatively young, an increase in the lower number represents an increase in the **vascular resistance** to blood flow. Thus an increase in vascular resistance is the first major reasons why blood pressure numbers go up.

Vascular resistance

This term refers to how hard it is to "push" the blood through the circulation. When resistance is high it takes more force to move blood through the tissues.

The second reason is more germane to the older patient and focuses on how elastic, or stretchable, the main arteries are. As we age, our blood vessels tend to lose their elasticity—that is, they stiffen, or harden, with age. When the heart beats to pump blood into these stiffer blood vessels, it takes more pressure to eject the blood from the heart and into the circulation, which is reflected by an increase in the upper number. Thus the blood pressure measurement, particularly when the person is older, indicates the interplay between stiffness and resistance. In younger people, resistance seems more important. In older people, stiffness seems more important.

As a person ages, the recoil in his or her blood vessels tends to become compromised, especially if the individual has high blood pressure for many years. The effect of this loss of recoil is that the lower number drifts down on its own sometime after the person's fiftieth birthday. Thus, if you graph the upper blood pressure number values in a population against the individuals' ages, the upper number values continue to increase until people die. A group of people who are 80 years old will, on average, have higher upper numbers than a group of people who are 60, or 40, or 20 years old. If you graph the lower blood pressure number values in a population against age, these values also rise until about age 50 to 55, after which they begin to fall. Consequently, the lower number in the blood pressure reading is more predictive of cardiovascular outcomes when you're younger, and the upper number is more predictive of cardiovascular outcomes when you're older. That relationship explains why physicians pay more attention to the upper number, particularly in older patients.

75. How does a doctor decide which medication to give to someone with high blood pressure?

Just as when a chef bakes a soufflé, a great deal of preparation and work go into the physician's choice of a medication for his or her patient with high blood pressure. Most doctors go through a checklist similar to this one when trying to come to that particular decision:

1. How old is this person?
2. What is this person's ethnic background?
3. Has there been any target organ damage in this person?
4. Are there other cardiovascular risk factors in this person?
5. Has this person been on blood pressure medicines in the past and, if so, were there any problems?
6. What other medications is the person taking, and are there any potential drug interactions that might cause worry?

In addition, financial considerations sometimes come into play. Not everyone has insurance or can afford the latest and most expensive blood pressure medications.

The blood pressure measurement indicates the interplay between stiffness and resistance. In younger people, resistance seems more important; in older people, stiffness seems more important. Thus the lower number in the blood pressure reading is more predictive of cardiovascular outcomes when you're younger, and the upper number is more predictive of cardiovascular outcomes when you're older.

If I were to simply prescribe any blood pressure medicine available, one or two times out of three the patient would probably experience a decent blood-pressure-lowering effect. Given this likelihood, the goal in managing someone's blood pressure is to do better than you would by just chance alone. By using the checklist given previously, physicians can typically prescribe a drug that yields a good blood pressure response in eight out of 10 patients.

Most patients' blood pressure can't be completely controlled with one medication, so physicians often have to choose a second drug for their patients.

The more challenging issue is that most patients' blood pressure can't be completely controlled with one medication. Only about four times out of 10 is a single agent successful in reducing blood pressure to less than 140/90 mm Hg. Thus physicians often have to choose a second drug for their patients. To do so, they go through the same kind of thinking pointed out in Figure 2 (see Question 14), trying to choose agents that have complementary (and not overlapping) mechanisms of action to lower blood pressure. Given this fact, I would add one more question to the checklist:

7. Does this medicine complement the other blood pressure medicine(s) the person is currently using?

PART FIVE

Physician/ Provider Issues

What do I do when different doctors tell me to take different medications?

When do I need to consult a hypertension specialist?

Should my doctor refer me to a cardiologist, a nephrologist, an endocrinologist, or some other specialist to help me get my blood pressure under control?

More . . .

76. What do I do when different doctors tell me to take different medications?

To continue the baking analogy used in Question 75, this question brings to mind the aphorism about too many cooks spoiling the broth. When you see multiple doctors, it's important to develop a "silo" approach.

For example, when you see your cholesterol doctor, the primary goal should be managing that aspect of your health. Naturally, your blood pressure may have been checked at your cholesterol-focused visit, and you might be nervous about your last blood cholesterol test given all those fancy dinners you had while you were hiring that new partner—so perhaps your blood pressure is a little higher than usual. If the doctor at that visit suggests that you take more blood pressure medication, he or she is clearly trying to act in your best interest. My patients will (I hope) politely inform other physicians that I am the one taking care of their blood pressure and that, while they appreciate the suggestion, they would rather talk this issue over with me first.

The only time this approach doesn't really work is when, for reasons that are sometimes not evident, your blood pressure is unusually high. In that case it's probably not safe to leave the problem unattended, or at least unchecked in terms of monitoring. If you cannot reach your blood pressure doctor to discuss the recommendations given by a different doctor, then you should follow those recommendations (when a safety issue is involved, such as unusually high blood pressure) until you can make contact with the person taking care of that aspect of your health.

Being a primary care physician can sometimes be bewildering when a patient with a variety of health conditions sees a group of subspecialists. Some of my patients have complained that they feel as if all they do is "see doctors." Some have as many as six or seven different medical doctors, each of whom the patient may visit once a month—or even more often depending on how sick the individual is. The challenge is to make sure that when you see any physician, you carry an accurate medication summary with you. Either take the pill bottles with you, or maintain an active list that contains all your drug names, the dose, the frequency with which you take it, and the point at which a new prescription will be needed. Sometimes the problem is that doctors don't appreciate that someone is taking a particular medication when they recommend something else be used. Moreover, some physicians will look at your medication regimen and conclude that they might not have done it that way and make a recommendation based on their own biases.

The most practical advice I can give you is this: Heed the recommendations of those healthcare providers in whom you have the most confidence. If you're unhappy with certain people who take care of you, let your primary care doctor know. There are many different subspecialists out there, and—as with medications—it's usually possible to find one in whom you have confidence.

Virginia comments:

I have a wonderful primary care doctor who coordinates my medications while bending to the advice of specialists to whom he has referred me. I am very vocal about medication preferences, and he is (thankfully) receptive to my wishes that are evidence-based (conclusions reached via clinical trials). Otherwise, I could not stick with a primary care doctor. Again, it's all about teamwork!

77. When do I need to consult a hypertension specialist?

There really aren't great guidelines for answering this particular question. I faced this challenge when I developed a module for the American College of Physicians to help

Heed the recommendations of those healthcare providers in whom you have the most confidence. If you're unhappy with certain people who take care of you, let your primary care doctor know.

Internal Medicine doctors manage blood pressure through a Web site-based education program called PIER. (Physicians Information and Education Resource) Here is the advice I gave them about when to consult a hypertension specialist:

- If blood pressure is not controlled after a year of trying
- If blood pressure is not controlled after three medications have been used at the same time
- If the doctor believes that a secondary hypertension may be present but is not sure how to proceed to evaluate or treat it
- If target organ damage is present, it sometimes helps to have that kind of subspecialist assist in blood pressure control

For example, if heart disease is present, a cardiologist may be able to both manage the heart disease and provide useful recommendations about blood pressure control. If kidney disease is present, a kidney doctor (nephrologist) can be quite useful in providing recommendations for both the kidney disease and blood pressure control.

78. Should my doctor refer me to a cardiologist, a nephrologist, an endocrinologist, or some other specialist to help me get my blood pressure under control?

Picking up the thread of discussion in Question 77, part of the issue may be availability in your area. Not everyone lives in a major urban center where numerous specialists are at the beck and call of your primary providing physician. In some locations, only a cardiologist or only a nephrologist who does hypertension consult care may be available. To answer the question more specifically, it does help to know whether there has been any cardiac or kidney or endocrine component in your history that might lead your doctor to choose one subspecialist over another.

In years gone by, much hypertension care was provided by cardiologists. The American Heart Association (AHA) recognized that fact, and today it operates a council devoted to high blood pressure and high blood pressure research. The U.S. guidelines for high blood pressure care are developed under the auspices of a federal agency, the National Heart, Lung, and Blood Institute of the National Institutes of Health (NIH). Clearly, there's quite a bit of track record of cardiologists managing high blood pressure.

By comparison, nephrologists often feel that they treat the patients with the most difficult-to-control kinds of high blood pressure. Moreover, these specialists tend to treat a population consisting of sick people and are used to managing patients who take a large number of medications.

When it comes to endocrinology, the relationship between diabetes and high blood pressure is well established. Consequently, endocrinologists are quite often exposed to patients with high blood pressure because they are often involved in diabetes care.

The moral of story: Your physician will likely know who does a good job at treating high blood pressure in area. Ask him or her for a referral if you need one.

79. What should I do if medication does not help my blood pressure?

As mentioned in Question 75, sometimes medicine just doesn't seem to do the job of reducing blood pressure. The culprit in such cases is often the servos (as discussed in Question 14 and illustrated in Figure 2). If you use a diuretic to treat the salt servo, for example, another aspect of the servo (such as the humoral side) may become much more active and trump the diuretic's ability to lower blood pressure. Conversely, if you choose a vasodilator first from the autoregulation servo, the salt servo may leap into action, causing you to retain salt and keeping your blood pressure from responding to the vasodilator. So what should you do?

When I lived in Texas between 1988 and 1993, I heard a Texas proverb that is applicable to this instance: "When your horse is dead, it's time to get off." There are times when you should simply give up medicine A and resort to medicine B. But it is important to check on a few things while you rummage around trying to find that optimal blood pressure medicine/patient marriage—namely, the lifestyle issues mentioned previously in several different questions. Some blood pressure medications simply will not work if you continue to consume large amounts of salt in your diet. If your medication isn't working, review the points in Question 23 and do your best to work on these issues while you also work on finding the best medication that works for you.

80. How can I have confidence that my doctor will listen to me if I have side effects?

Some of my friends tell me I rush in where fools fear to tread, but here goes: Doctors belong to a profession whose primary goal is to help people feel better and take care of themselves. When we prescribe a medication and the patient experiences a side effect, sometimes we internalize that result and feel as if we were somehow responsible for the "failure." This may happen unconsciously, but it makes us wonder if we made the right choice. Then our ego springs into action, defending our choice and making other rationalizations. The net effect is that some doctors accept side effects as a fact of life, knowing that they are likely to happen and being prepared to respond when needed. Other physicians think that patients read too much and that pharmacists give out too much literature about side effects—we're doctors, and we know better. Those doctors may not be quite as ready to acknowledge that a patient has a legitimate complaint. People are people, and it takes all kinds to make up a healthcare system.

So what can you do? First, you can be as specific as possible when covering the issue. You'll get more traction if you can pinpoint exactly what you feel and provide some sense of when it happens and how much it disturbs your quality of life. Health care is a service industry, and the members of this profession are here to serve you. We can do that best when we have a good handle on just what is happening to a person who is experiencing side effects. A report of "That pill makes me sick" is not very helpful. A complaint of "I get a headache most afternoons that starts around two or three o'clock" is much more useful: Now the physician has something that he or she can track. Also, if your medication changes, you and your physician will know what to look for in the future.

Second, you should keep an open mind. Not everything that you feel is automatically related to the medication that you take. When other explanations for symptoms are possible, be prepared to at least hear that they may be the cause. For example, sometimes that pain in your knees is really **osteoarthritis,** and not the blood pressure medicine.

Third, take a personal inventory and ask yourself honestly, "How many medications have I taken that have caused me to have side effects?" If the answer is "Just about all of them," it may be extremely difficult to find a drug you can tolerate. Some people have multiple chemical sensitivities, which makes it nearly impossible to treat them without a great deal of trial and error. In a busy office practice, it can be challenging to devote a large amount of time to an individual patient when someone has these kinds of medication-tolerance problems. One option that may be feasible is to try to be the last appointment of the day. *Sometimes* the lack of other waiting patients will help ensure that you have enough time to be heard by your doctor.

When discussing side effects of your medications with your healthcare provider, keep three guidelines in mind: Be specific, keep an open mind, and take a personal inventory first.

Osteoarthritis
Inflammation and stiffness of the joints that usually occurs in older persons as a result of deterioration of the cartilage around the joints.

81. What kinds of tests do I routinely need for my high blood pressure care?

Physicians perform three basic kinds of tests routinely when caring for someone with high blood pressure: an electrocardiogram, blood tests, and urine tests.

An electrocardiogram is a kind of a tape recording that shows how your heart is doing from an electrical viewpoint. It is used for two purposes:

- To check for thickening of the heart muscle
- To diagnose a heart attack that may or may not have been accompanied by symptoms

When a heart attack occurs without the symptoms being recognized by a person, it is called a silent heart attack. These events are more common in people with diabetes, but also occur in people without diabetes.

The second kind of test performed in patients with hypertension is a series of blood evaluations. These tests measure kidney function, blood sugar, the lipid panel, the body's mineral balance, and usually the amount of hemoglobin in the blood:

- Kidney function may change as a result of target organ damage from high blood pressure. This change would be manifested in a blood test that measures the amount of creatinine. Creatinine is a waste product, and its levels in the blood rise when the kidney function becomes impaired.
- Blood sugar is monitored to identify the development of diabetes. This gets at an issue mentioned earlier: Does the person have cardiovascular risk factors that, in conjunction with hypertension, put him or her at risk for having heart disease or stroke in the future? (See Question 87.)
- The lipid panel quantifies the amounts of cholesterol and triglycerides present in the body. Their levels are very important to watch in someone who is at risk for heart disease and stroke owing to the presence of hypertension.
- The body's mineral balance is monitored because sometimes medications affect the levels of sodium and

potassium in the blood. In the case of low potassium, it may be necessary to give the patient a potassium supplement.

- It is important to measure the amount of hemoglobin in the blood because very high levels of hemoglobin make the blood thicker and contribute to elevated blood pressure levels.

The third kind of testing performed on patients with hypertension focuses on three components of the urine: blood, protein and sugar. Abnormal blood and protein levels may reflect damage to the kidney, or they may indicate that something is happening in the kidney that may predispose the person to hypertension or worsen his or her blood pressure control. The measurement of sugar in the urine simply serves as a check on diabetes; it is a little redundant given that the blood tests check the level of sugar as well. All three urine-based tests are done on a single stick called a dipstick, and they typically take only a minute to do.

In my practice, I tend to perform an electrocardiogram every 2 to 4 years in someone who is younger and has relatively low cardiovascular risk. In someone who is older than age 55, an electrocardiogram done yearly or every 2 years would be reasonable. I encourage my patients to have the blood tests once a year, with the urine dipstick being performed at the same time.

82. My doctor ordered an arteriogram of my kidneys. Is that dangerous?

An **arteriogram** is a test in which x-ray dye is injected down each of the kidney arteries to look for blockages. When blockages are present, the person is said to have **renal** vascular disease. Most such blockages are caused by longstanding high blood pressure, cigarette smoking, and high levels of cholesterol. Not uncommonly, all three of these factors are present in a person who has renal vascular disease. Your physician may listen

Arteriogram

A medical procedure in which dye is injected into a blood vessel. This is done to identify narrowing or to define an important aspect of anatomy such as presence of a tumor or a swelling (aneurysm) of the blood vessel.

Renal

Pertaining to the kidney.

over the kidney arteries in your upper stomach area for bruits (pronounced "broo-eeze"), which are the noises that blood makes when it's flowing through areas of blockage. Kidney artery blockage may be suspected when someone has the three factors mentioned previously (hypertension, cigarettes, high cholesterol), bruits, and kidney function that's below the normal range.

One of the most common reasons that an arteriogram is performed is the fact that high blood pressure is very hard to control in some people who are thought to have renal vascular disease. In some people, correcting the narrowing in the kidney artery improves blood pressure control.

All arteriograms are associated with a certain amount of risk. The radiologist or cardiologist who performs the arteriogram must first puncture an artery to enable a catheter to be maneuvered to the place where the arteriogram can be done. In the case of the kidneys, the insertion is usually done in the leg at the level of the groin. As the catheter is advanced from the groin up to the level of the kidney arteries, the physician may discover that the big artery (the aorta) has a lot of atherosclerotic disease. In such a case, the lining of the aorta (which should normally be smooth) may be shaggy and studded with cholesterol crystals, which can be shaved off as the catheter is advanced past segments that have these kinds of plaques. The small crystals, once broken off, act like torpedoes and can impact in areas such as the skin, toes, intestines, or kidneys and cause troubles. Fortunately, the physicians doing these procedures are very well aware of this possibility and take precautions to minimize the likelihood that it will happen. This complication occurs in only about 1% of all arteriograms.

More common is the development of a bruise at the arterial puncture site. These wounds can be very small—in fact, almost unnoticeable. When the patient's blood pressure is very high or he or she takes blood-thinning medicines, however, the bruises may be bigger. Occasionally, these patients have some discomfort at the bruised site.

When you go for the arteriogram, you will be asked to sign a consent form. If you think that the package inserts that come with your bottles of medication can be scary, be aware that the consent form can sometimes outdo these warnings! Keep in mind that the consent form has to be written in such a way as to encompass any and every possibility of harm. The professionals who perform these procedures have typically been doing them for a long time, however, and they will take many precautions to ensure that you will be as safe and as comfortable as possible during the procedure.

83. I have heard that an operation on the neck can improve high blood pressure. What is that about?

A company called CVRx is currently studying a device, called the Rheos system, that works much like a pacemaker but is attached to the carotid artery in the neck instead of the heart. Remember our old friend the baroreceptor (see Question 36)? Once again, the baroreceptor takes center stage for this question. The new device paces the baroreceptor; that is, it basically convinces the baroreceptor that the blood pressure is at a higher level than it should be. As a consequence, the baroreceptor sends responses to the involuntary nervous system center in the brain telling it to "cool down" and lower the blood pressure.

The Rheos system is still in the experimental stages. So far it's mostly been used in people whose blood pressure has failed to come down on conventional blood pressure medicines. Its use requires an operation where small electrodes are placed on the surface of the carotid artery, a wire is passed under the skin to the chest, and the wire is then connected to a box about the size of the pacemaker, which is placed under the skin in the upper chest. Once the surgical wound has healed, then the box is programmed to pace the baroreceptor at the optimal level that reduces blood pressure. Although the data for the Rheos system are only preliminary at this point, the device seems to work well and apparently continues to work for at least one to two years after implantation.

84. My upper arm is relatively large, so my doctor takes my blood pressure near my wrist. Is that accurate?

If your blood pressure is taken under the conditions described in Question 8, then even a measurement of the blood pressure taken in the wrist is likely to be accurate. Some people have what's called a funnel-shaped arm—that is, the circumference of the arm at the shoulder is much larger than the circumference of the arm just above the elbow. Using even large adult cuffs to take someone's blood pressure can be very difficult in these circumstances, because the cuffs tend to slip down and the Velcro doesn't hold well. Moreover, the cuffs may not compress the arm correctly and could grossly overestimate the true blood pressure.

Taking the blood pressure at the wrist gets around the problems with the upper arm geometry. There are some concerns about how accurate the wrist blood pressure is, but the inaccuracy—if any—is probably small (in the range of 3 to 4 mm Hg).

There are two ways to take the blood pressure at the level of the wrist. One way is to take the measurement the same way you normally do on the upper arm, by pumping up the cuff on the forearm and then listening with a stethoscope over the artery at the wrist on the thumb side. This is tricky, and not all doctors have been trained in doing this kind of procedure. The alternative, which is far more common, is to use one of the digital blood pressure kits. This situation is one circumstance where it helps to take multiple readings, particularly after a good five-minute rest period. If this practice produces two or three relatively close readings, odds are they're pretty good. I have treated several patients based only on wrist blood pressures and they certainly seem to do okay.

85. My doctor ordered an echocardiogram. How will that help her take care of my high blood pressure?

An **echocardiogram** uses sound waves to take a picture of the heart. It can tell us several very important things about how someone's heart is doing when that person has high blood pressure. For example, it can reveal how thick the heart walls are, which is important in determining the extent of success in controlling the blood pressure. When we do a good job controlling the blood pressure, usually the heart walls are within normal thickness range.

An echocardiogram can also indicate whether the heart has sustained any damage. It do so in one of two ways. The first way is a reduction in the ejection fraction. The ejection fraction is a measure of how efficiently the heart beats each time it goes through one of its cycles. A normal ejection fraction is 50% to 55% (or higher). The second way is by looking at how all the parts of the heart wall work during each heartbeat when the heart contracts. In a normal heart, all segments contract equally at the same time. In a heart that has sustained damage, some segments do not contract as forcefully or may not even move at all when the rest of the heart is beating.

In addition, the echocardiogram provides information about pulmonary hypertension if this condition is present. Normally the pulmonary (lung) circulation operates under much lower pressure than the values we typically see when we measure blood pressure in the arm. Elevated levels of pressure in the pulmonary circulation are sometimes very difficult to suspect on clinical grounds.

Physicians order echocardiograms when they suspect there may be heart involvement from high blood pressure based, for example, on the electrocardiogram. They may also order an echocardiogram when they're concerned that someone who

---

Echocardiogram

A sound wave test that provides a picture of the heart. It usually gives a measure of heart wall thickness, how well the valves work and how efficiently the heart contracts.

Physician/Provider Issues

appears to have white-coat hypertension (see Question 11) may actually be experiencing more of a blood pressure load than suspected. In this circumstance, the physician looks for early signs of high blood pressure affecting the heart muscle. These signs are quite subtle and are not usually evident on electrocardiogram or even on physical exam. In other circumstances, doctors order echocardiograms to pursue heart murmurs, which they may hear when they listen to the chest, or gallop sounds, which are extra sounds that the heart sometimes makes in case of high blood pressure or heart failure (these sounds resemble a horse's hoof beats—hence the name).

86. I had an electrocardiogram at my hypertension visit today. The doctor said it wasn't exactly normal but that it was okay for someone with high blood pressure like me. What did that mean?

I have said those exact words to many patients over the years. There are three kinds of electrocardiogram findings: clearly normal, clearly abnormal, and all the rest. This kind of question was asked by someone whose cardiogram fell into the "all the rest" category. To understand the doctor's response, it may help to know what exactly an electrocardiogram does and why this is such a common finding.

An electrocardiogram measures the electrical activity of the heart, but it cannot tell how well the heart is beating. If the doctor wants to understand the heart function, he or she usually orders an echocardiogram.

An electrocardiogram measures the electrical activity of the heart, but it doesn't know beans about how *well* the heart is beating. In other words, it simply makes an electrical recording and makes no claims whatsoever about the actual heart function. If the doctor wants to understand the heart function, he or she must order an echocardiogram. Echocardiograms cost loads more than electrocardiograms, so doctors usually make do with the electrocardiogram and use the echocardiogram only in selected circumstances (see Question 85).

The electrocardiogram looks at the heart from about 12 different angles, which we call leads, leading to clever terminology like "a 12-lead electrocardiogram." The little squiggles on the paper represent the upper and lower parts of the heart, which beat in sequence. Most of the problems occur with the last part of the electrocardiogram, a segment known as the T wave. A nice, healthy T wave is usually upright. When the T wave is flat, or upside down, it may just be a variant of normal and has uncertain significance. The medical term for this phenomenon is nonspecific S-T and T wave changes; see **Figure 4.**

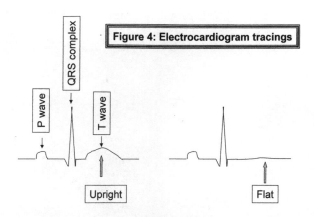

Figure 4: Electrocardiogram tracings

Legend: On the left is a normal electrical representation of a heartbeat. On the right the T wave is flattened; this is considered a "non-specific" finding.

Figure 4   Electrocardiogram tracings

Nonspecific S-T and T wave changes are not considered normal, but they are also not considered clearly abnormal; rather, they fall somewhere in between. The word "nonspecific" tells the whole story: It means that something may be up, but we are not sure what. While people with high blood pressure often show these changes, so do people without high blood pressure. As far as we know, there is no particularly ominous aspect to nonspecific S-T and T wave changes. For that reason, physicians don't usually change therapy or worry excessively when we see these changes.

PART SIX

Other Health Problems/ Issues

Why do my blood pressure readings have to be even lower than the readings for other people with hypertension when I have diabetes?

I have bad allergies. What can I take for them that will not interfere with my blood pressure?

How does high blood pressure affect the kidneys? How would I know if I had kidney damage?

More . . .

87. Why do my blood pressure readings have to be even lower than the readings for other people with hypertension when I have diabetes?

The current level of optimal blood pressure treatment is levels lower than 130/80 mm Hg for diabetics.

Several organizations, including the American Diabetes Association, the American Heart Association, and the National Kidney Foundation, have all come out with similar recommendations regarding the degree of blood pressure control that we should aim for in patients with diabetes. The current level of optimal blood pressure treatment is lower than 130/80 mm Hg for diabetics. This recommendation is based on findings from several research studies that included diabetics who had high blood pressure.

Both diabetes and high blood pressure are models of premature aging of the circulation. Thus, when both are present, there is the potential for even more hardening of the arteries at a younger age. When research studies on high blood pressure therapy have been done in patients with diabetes, their results have clearly shown that greater blood pressure reduction translates into greater target organ preservation. Some experts argue that the recommended level of 130/80 mm Hg in patients with diabetes should actually be even lower, and some say it should be as low as 110/70 mm Hg.

Some research suggests that when diabetes is present, it is akin to having known coronary artery blockage; thus the medical literature includes statements like "Diabetes is a coronary artery disease equivalent." Of the many different disorders that can coexist with high blood pressure, diabetes is the one circumstance where blood pressure reduction pays off the best in terms of keeping the heart, brain, and kidneys working for a longer period of time. This feat comes at no small cost to the patient, however. Getting blood pressures down below the 130/80 mm Hg level can be challenging, often taking three or more drugs to achieve this goal.

88. I have bad allergies. What can I take for them that will not interfere with my blood pressure?

Plain antihistamines, although they may be sedating, usually do not wreak havoc on your blood pressure. They are considered safe for most patients with hypertension.

Decongestants are another story. Most decongestants, whether obtained by prescription or bought over the counter, contain warnings about their usage in patients with high blood pressure. The danger arises because decongestants work like adrenaline, acting on the adrenergic servo (see Figure 2 in Question 14), and doing the opposite of medications such as alpha blockers. In fact, one of the side effects of alpha blockers is a stuffy nose sensation. When decongestants are absolutely needed, I ask my patients to take only short-acting ones (*not* the 12- or 24-hour versions) and to use these medications only when they are in dire straits.

Another option is to see an allergist to obtain shots that desensitize you to allergens. These kinds of shots don't usually raise blood pressure, and they may afford relief if you are a viable candidate for this kind of therapy.

89. How does high blood pressure affect the kidneys? How would I know if I had kidney damage?

The kidney has been called both a victim and the villain in hypertension. It is a *victim* in that the kidney is one of the target organs that can be damaged by high blood pressure. It is a *villain* in that the kidney may contribute to elevated blood pressure by retaining salt, thereby causing blood pressure to go up through this servo. Let's talk about the victim aspect first.

While the heart and brain get most of the attention as the target organs that are damaged by high blood pressure, high blood pressure clearly damages the kidneys of some people. In this regard, there is a remarkable difference in the likelihood of hypertension-related kidney damage depending on ethnic background. For reasons that are still largely not explained, patients of African American descent tend to have the most damage to their kidneys from high blood pressure; they are four to six times more likely to experience kidney damage from high blood pressure compared with white patients.

The kidney circulation has some amazing features. For instance, it is very responsive to changes in the blood pressure level because the kidney must clear wastes from the blood around the clock. Because it has to do its work under all kinds of blood pressure levels, the kidney's remarkable system of arteries must adapt to the many changes in blood pressure that are typical in the course of the day. One unique characteristic of the kidney is a set of filter units called **glomeruli,** which are very much like spaghetti colanders. The glomeruli allow the fluid portion of blood to be filtered out (like separating the water from the spaghetti), but they retain the proteins and cells such as red blood cells, white blood cells, and platelets in the blood (like holding back the spaghetti). The glomeruli are protected from the brunt of high levels of blood pressure by the circulation upwind of them. In some people, however, this upwind circulation doesn't work as well, which exposes their glomeruli to higher blood pressures leading to damage and ultimately their destruction. This outcome is particularly likely in African American patients and in diabetics.

Glomeruli

These are the tiny filter units in each kidney that initiate the formation of urine. In health they allow only the liquid part of blood to be filtered, and a barrier against protein or cells like red blood cells appearing in the urine.

As to the role of villain, the kidney is the main regulator of the body's salt servo balance (see Figure 2 in Question 14). In addition, the kidney is the major source of renin, one of the humoral servo compounds that raises blood pressure (see Figure 2). Both angiotensin-converting enzyme (ACE) inhibitors and angiotensin-receptor-blocking drugs are given to reduce the effects of the renin system. Some research also suggests that patients with kidney damage have higher levels of adrenergic servo activity. Through at least three different ways, then, the kidney can participate in raising blood pressure and maintaining the hypertensive state.

Very often kidney damage occurs without any particular sign or symptom indicating its presence. There are a few things to pay attention to that will help you be aware of whether you have, or are predisposed to, kidney damage. The most important thing is to have your creatinine checked regularly (see Question 81). The other thing to know is whether you have a close relative who has experienced kidney damage, been on dialysis, or needed a kidney transplant. This fact would give you a family history of kidney disease and should put you on your guard to watch your own kidney function carefully. Lastly, if you have ever told by a healthcare worker that you have blood or protein in your urine, it would be important to follow up on that information; these components in the urine may be early markers of kidney damage or signs that your kidney may be contributing to elevated levels of blood pressure.

Very often kidney damage occurs without any particular sign or symptom indicating its presence.

90. How did the eye doctor know by looking into my eyes that I have high blood pressure?

When the doctor looks into your eyes, he or she is looking at the back part of your eye—the area known as the retina. When you look at the retina, you can actually see little tiny arteries and little tiny veins, which are called arterioles and veinules, respectively. In healthy people, there is a well-known relationship between the caliber, or size, of the arteriole and the veinule. When hypertension is present, this relationship changes because the arteriole is more constricted, or smaller. The result is called grade 1 changes or grade 1 **retinopathy.**

Normally the blood vessels in the retina criss-cross somewhat. In healthy people, the criss-crossings look perfectly normal. In people with hypertension, when the arteriole crosses over

Retinopathy

Pertaining to harmful effects in the back of the eye (i.e. the retina).

in front of the veinule, it pinches the veinule, producing a characteristic look called nicking. The result is called grade 2 retinopathy.

In patients with more severe elevations in blood pressure, particularly when these elevations have been present for a while, little areas of the retina may have experienced a form of gangrene called infarction. The affected areas are called cotton-wool spots because they look white and fluffy like old-fashioned cotton-wool. The other finding at this stage, grade 3 retinopathy, consists of small bleeding spots, which sometimes look like tiny fires and are called flame hemorrhages. See **Figure 5.**

Optic

Pertaining to the eye.

Pappiledema

Swelling of the place in the eye where the nerves and blood supply of the retina enter the eye from the brain.

The eyes are really an extension of the brain, and in the back of the eye is a small area called the **optic** cup where the optic nerve connects from the eyes directly to the brain. Normally this cup has a sharp border or rim. The most severe form of high blood pressure affecting the eye, which is called **pappiledema** or grade 4 retinopathy, results in a blurring of this usually sharp cup border. When doctors see these kinds of changes, they send patients directly to the hospital, usually calling ahead to make sure that they are seen quickly because this usually is a true medical emergency.

How do we know so much about the relationship between hypertension and the eyes? In the 1930s, when no effective blood pressure medication was available, one of the more important steps that was taken to evaluate the severity of a patient's high blood pressure was to look carefully into his or her eyes. An elaborate classification scheme based on the appearance of the retinal circulation was developed that predicted relatively accurately which patients were likely to have only modest changes in their longevity (grade 1 or 2) versus which patients might have less than one year to live (grade 4). Nowadays, of course, it's far less common to see cotton-wool spots, flame hemorrhages, and pappiledema.

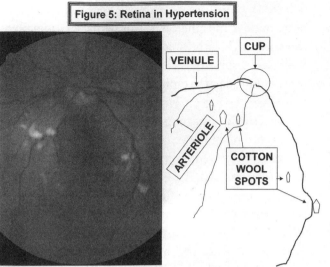

Figure 5: Retina in Hypertension

VEINULE

CUP

ARTERIOLE

COTTON WOOL SPOTS

Used with permission from Mohler and Townsend - Advanced Therapy in Hypertension and Vascular Disease. 2006. B. C. Dekker publishers

Legend: On left is a real picture of the retina. On right is a cartoon showing the arteriole and veinule sizes, and cotton wool spots (the little pentagons).

Figure 5   Retina in hypertension. Used with permission from Mohler and Townsend. Advanced Therapy in Hypertension and Vascular Disease. B.C. Decker, Inc., 2006.

91. If I have had a heart attack, does that mean I should be taking special blood pressure medications?

The answer to this question is yes most of the time. Just which medication is prescribed is based on the recommendations for care developed by National Heart, Lung, and Blood Institute of the National Institutes of Health (NIH) and will depend somewhat on whether the heart attack was complicated. The guidelines for hypertension care are reevaluated every four or five years. This analysis has revealed that certain patients are best treated with specific classes of blood pressure medications. These circumstances are known as compelling indications, meaning that there is good evidence that we should use these drugs whenever possible in these particular situations.

Now, how about that issue with complications? When a heart attack occurs, it may or may not be complicated by heart failure. The heart attack in itself does some damage to the heart muscle. In some cases, this damage is enough to cause shortness of breath, tiredness, and sometimes leg swelling; this level of severity is called heart failure. In the absence of heart failure, doctors typically prescribe beta blockers, angiotensin-converting enzyme (ACE) inhibitors, and/or **mineralocorticoid** antagonists (MRAs) to their patients with hypertension who have suffered a heart attack. When heart failure has occurred, they still prescribe beta blockers, ACE inhibitors, and MRAs, but often add diuretics to the drug regimen to control the tendency toward fluid retention that is so characteristic of heart failure.

Mineralocorticoid

This term pertains to the salt, or mineral, retaining effects of adrenal cortical (see Cortex) hormones like aldosterone.

There are exceptions to these guidelines because some people really aren't good candidates for one or the other of these classes of medications. The general thinking goes like this:

- Beta blockers appear to reduce the risk of sudden cardiac death in the years after a heart attack.
- ACE inhibitors appear to preserve (and perhaps improve) what's left of the heart's normal architecture and may reduce the tendency toward heart failure in the future.
- MRAs may help reduce scarring, which appears to be a particular problem in heart failure because of the activation of many factors in the bloodstream and tissues that promote the formation of scarring in the vessels and in the heart itself.
- Angiotensin-receptor blockers are often used in place of ACE inhibitors (because of the side effects associated with ACE inhibitors, such as cough), although sometimes they are added on to a regimen that includes an ACE inhibitor as well.

Other medications are prescribed on a case-by-case basis to deal with specific symptoms that may occur in a patient who has had a heart attack or a heart attack complicated by heart failure. These drugs may include blood thinners, lipid medications, and vitamins such as folic acid and other dietary supplements that may help depending on the findings from your blood tests. Still other medications may be needed just to control your blood pressure, so don't be surprised if you are asked to take a calcium-channel blocker or some other medication for your hypertension.

92. I have an appointment for same-day surgery. What should I do about my blood pressure medications on that day?

The usual approach in this situation is to take your medications just as you normally do on the day of surgery with a couple of sips of water. Many times we ask people not to take their diuretic pill on the day of, and sometimes for one or two days prior to, surgery. This practice is a holdover from the time when low potassium values were very common in patients taking diuretics because we used larger doses of these medications in the past. Low potassium is rarely a problem now, but unless you hear otherwise, it's okay to skip your diuretic on the day of surgery.

Most times you will meet with someone from the anesthesia department prior to your appointment for surgery. This meeting would be a good time to discuss this matter, to make sure the anesthesiologist knows that you do take blood pressure medicines, and to confirm that he or she is okay with you taking your medications with a small amount of water on the day of your surgical procedure. The key is *not* to consume 12 full ounces of water. Usually the anesthesiologist wants your stomach to be empty because anesthesia sometimes produces nausea and you're more likely to have an episode of vomiting if your stomach is filled.

Some other medications may be discontinued around the time of the surgical procedure—namely, blood thinners in general, and aspirin in particular. Check with your doctors about these medications; they will often request that aspirin be stopped for at least a week before surgery is performed. People who take the blood thinner warfarin (brand name: Coumadin) need to have a good talk with both their medical doctors and their surgeons about how to handle this particular situation because it sometimes necessitates the use of an intravenous blood thinner called heparin around the time of surgery.

It's usually safe to restart your medicines once you are allowed to have a full liquid diet. At this point you usually have sounds in your stomach area that indicate your bowels are working again, and you should be able to tolerate medication from that point onward.

93. If I have had a stroke, will treating my blood pressure prevent another stroke from happening?

One of the more sobering statistics in medicine is that once a person has had a stroke, he or she has an approximately 20% chance of having another stroke in the next five years. High blood pressure is one of the leading risk factors for having a stroke someday, and stroke is the third leading cause of death in the United States, behind heart disease (number 1) and cancer (number 2). Of all the outcomes you can expect from treating high blood pressure with medication, a reduction in stroke incidence is one of the best-documented benefits. Once you have had a stroke, however, it doesn't mean that you have lost the battle and should give up. Plenty of good evidence indicates that you can still reduce your chances of experiencing a future stroke by treating your hypertension with medication. Some strokes are caused by irregularities in the heart rhythm, and people with this condition are usually treated with some kind of blood thinner in addition to blood pressure medications.

One combination of blood pressure medications that is promoted for treating someone who has already had a stroke is a combination of a diuretic and an angiotensin-converting enzyme (ACE) inhibitor. This combination was tested several years ago in a study called PROGRESS (Perindopril Protection Against Recurrent Stroke Study). In this study, the combination of diuretic and ACE inhibitor was given to patients whether or not they had hypertension (many participants did have elevated blood pressure). Interestingly, both individuals with hypertension and those without hypertension realized a benefit in terms of future stroke occurrence when both drugs were given together. There is a lot of interest in other combinations of blood pressure medications that might be used to prevent the next stroke, although less research has been done on these options to date. Such studies are now under way, and we should have a better handle on these combinations' benefits in a few years.

94. Why did my dentist tell me she could not do my dental work because my blood pressure needs to be better controlled before she could numb my tooth?

When dentists inject anesthesia so that they can work on their patients' teeth, they use a mixture of a numbing medication along with adrenaline. They do this because the numbing medication, when used alone, tends to get washed out of the tissues by the circulation and could potentially wear off before they finish their work. When adrenaline is added to these local anesthetics, they last much longer.

However, the patient does absorb the adrenaline, too. In most people, the absorption rate is rather slow and the consequences on their heart rate and blood pressure are trivial. We recently performed a study to measure the blood pressure changes in healthy people after a relatively sizable amount of adrenaline and local anesthetic was injected into the jaw, simulating the wisdom tooth extraction type of dental work. When we measured blood pressure at about 10-minute intervals, we observed a rise in the upper number of the blood pressure reading and the heart rate; this increase had mostly disappeared 20 minutes after the injection, and not too much happened after that.

In young healthy people, like those in this research study, there appears to be no health consequence from the adrenaline/anesthetic combination. In older people with high blood pressure or those with heart disease such as **angina,** however, the small rise in blood pressure and the small increase in heart rate could produce some symptoms—for example, chest discomfort. For that reason, dentists and oral surgeons prefer to see good blood pressure levels in patients who need to have their jaws numbed for dental work. The risks to any one person are probably small, but most dental problems are not life-threatening in themselves and it's considered prudent to ensure that someone's blood pressure is okay before exposing them to the risk associated with even a small amount of adrenaline.

Angina

A symptom of squeezing-type chest discomfort, often associated with physical exertion, that is associated with coronary artery blockage. The activity places extra demands on the heart and the blocked coronary circulation cannot supply the heart enough oxygen and nutrient to keep up which causes the 'ache' perceived as chest discomfort.

95. I am a young woman with hypertension who needs to be treated with medicine, but I also want to get pregnant. Which blood pressure medicines should I avoid? Are there any "safe" medicines in pregnancy?

Most of what we know about treating hypertension in someone who is young, female, and capable of becoming pregnant comes from case-control studies. In this kind of study someone with a problem or issue (a 'case') is matched up with someone without the problem or issue (a 'control'). In the past, it was usually considered good science to compare active treatment to placebo tablets and to include large numbers of mostly older people with high blood pressure in research studies. By contrast, the idea of doing this kind of randomized controlled study in women who could become pregnant or who are already pregnant, and who have hypertension, would raise such huge ethical barriers that such an investigation is unlikely to be done at this time. So what do we know?

Other Health Problems/Issues

At least two classes of antihypertensive medications carry the dreaded "black box warning." That is, the package inserts for these drugs—which detail everything you ever wanted to know about these medications—must include an area enclosed in a black box that warns the potential consumer (and the prescribing doctor) about the risks of the medicine when it is used during pregnancy. The two classes of blood pressure medications that doctors try to avoid prescribing in pregnancy are angiotensin-converting enzyme (ACE) inhibitors and angiotensin-receptor blockers. Evidence suggests that ACE inhibitors are not good for the developing child; specifically, these medications have been shown to impair bone development and kidney maturation in the developing child. We have less evidence about angiotensin-receptor blockers, but they are felt to be related to ACE inhibitors and are "guilty by association."

The story about diuretics in pregnancy has gone back and forth over the years. At one time diuretics were frequently used to control the ankle swelling that often happens normally in pregnancy. Rare consequences of diuretic use for the unborn child include being small for gestational age owing to blood flow problems with the placenta, problems with bilirubin (the chemical that causes jaundice or yellow skin in babies and adults), and low platelets.

Beta blockers, calcium-channel blockers, alpha$_2$ agonists (such as methyldopa [trade name: Aldomet]), and the vasodilator hydralazine (trade name: Apressoline) are all believed to be reasonably safe in pregnancy. There's not much evidence that they cause harm, and all of these medications can be effective in controlling blood pressure in the expectant hypertensive mother when needed.

Even when the mother's and fetus' care is in the best of obstetrical hands, there's always a certain low incidence of birth defects (approximately 1% or 2% of births). These problems can be innocuous, such as a red spot on the baby's

Beta blockers, calcium-channel blockers, alpha$_2$ agonists, and hydralazine are believed to be reasonably safe in pregnancy. ACE inhibitors and angiotensin-receptor blockers should be avoided in pregnant women.

forearm, or serious, such as a cleft palate. When a woman takes no medications during her pregnancy, these defects are typically blamed on genetic disorders of one kind or another, or another cause or explanation is sought. When a woman takes medication during pregnancy, it always raises the possibility that the medication may have influenced the birth defect. There are some well-documented examples in which medications have caused abnormalities in the developing child. For example, use of the drug thalidomide in the 1950s resulted in children being born with flippers instead of hands or feet, a phenomenon called phocomelia. No such sensational effects have been found with the beta blockers, calcium-channel blockers, alpha$_2$ agonists, or hydralazine, and most obstetricians, primary care doctors, and high-risk obstetrical hypertension specialists use them to manage hypertension in pregnancy.

96. I am nursing my new baby now. Which medications can I take for my blood pressure while nursing?

The classes of medications mentioned in Question 95 (i.e., beta blockers, calcium-channel blockers, alpha$_2$ agonists, and hydralazine) are sometimes continued even into the nursing period. There have been some attempts to document how much medication is eliminated from the body through breast milk. This research is limited, however, so doctors often rely just on their own clinical experience to guide them in this circumstance.

In general, nursing continues for six to 12 months before the baby is weaned. Most drugs, when excreted in breast milk, are in fairly low concentrations; thus the baby doesn't get a full adult dose of medication. How much gets into the milk, which is known as the milk/plasma (M/P) ratio, depends on the medication itself and its ability to stick to the proteins that usually carry drugs in the liquid part of the blood (i.e., the plasma). There is significant variability in the rates at which drugs are secreted into the breast milk, and a child could experience blood pressure and heart rate changes from absorbing too much of an antihypertensive drug while breastfeeding. Thus this issue is a cause for concern.

A group of scientists from Australia assembled the available information on this topic in an article published in 2002. (You can see the abstract of their article by going to http://www.pubmed.com and typing in the reference number 12044345 in the blank white box in the opening page.) Here's what they said, in a nutshell:

The available data to date indicate that ACE inhibitors, methyldopa, beta blockers with high protein binding, and some calcium-channel blockers all appear to be safe treatments of hypertension in a nursing mother. The data suggest that drugs to be avoided are beta blockers with low protein binding. However, the available evidence is limited and further studies are needed to confirm these findings.

There is also a web site that addresses the passage of drugs into breast milk, as noted in the "Literature and Other Sources of Information" appendix at the end of this book.

97. My doctor was very concerned about finding protein in my urine. What is the significance of that?

Finding protein in the urine—a condition called **proteinuria**—is abnormal. The filtering units in the kidney (discussed in Question 89) are designed to keep proteins and cells inside the circulation and to let only water, minerals, and waste products pass through and become urine. When protein is detectable in the urine, it signals that this barrier in the glomeruli has been breached. One of the most common causes for this finding is diabetes. Many other circumstances can also affect the filtering units of the kidney and cause proteinuria.

Proteinuria

This term refers to the presence of protein in the urine. Protein is not usually detected in the urine healthy individuals.

Doctors see proteinuria as cause for concern because it is considered a sign that more than just a kidney issue is present. In particular, the risks of cardiovascular diseases such as stroke are deemed higher because proteinuria is believed to be a marker of a more general problem with the circulation. It is sometimes possible to adjust your medicines to reduce or even eliminate proteinuria. It is also possible that a cause for this condition can be found and potentially treated or removed. Several medications have the potential to increase urine protein excretion, so one of the first things doctors do when they find proteinuria is to review the patient's medication history.

Proteinuria may also be a sign of an underlying kidney problem, such as kidney damage from hypertension. Sometimes it is a marker of a problem that has arisen primarily within the kidney—for example, the filtering units might appear to have some kind of allergic reaction to something to which the person has been exposed. Besides predicting events such as stroke, proteinuria is one of the more important factors that affects why and how rapidly kidney failure progresses in some people. Higher levels of proteinuria are associated with a faster loss of kidney function over time.

When urinary protein is present but the doctor can't find any obvious cause for it, he or she typically orders blood and urine tests, and sometimes an imaging procedure (such as an ultrasound) of the kidneys to look for the source of the excess protein. In some cases, when the urine protein losses are very high, a kidney **biopsy** may be performed to determine precisely what the problem is and to decide whether it can be managed with medications. In some cases, the medications used to treat proteinuria are similar to the drugs used in cancer care or to maintain the function of transplanted organs. These drugs can be heavy hitters, so it's important to be sure of the diagnosis before starting a patient on one. Although a kidney biopsy has some definite risks associated with it, the benefits of knowing what's going on usually outweigh its drawbacks.

Proteinuria is considered a sign that more than just a kidney issue is present. It may be possible to adjust anti-hypertensive medications to reduce or even eliminate proteinuria or to identify and treat another underlying cause.

Biopsy

A piece of tissue removed from the body and examined for abnormalities.

98. My mother had hypertension caused by some kind of tumor in her adrenal gland. Should my doctor look for a tumor in me?

If you take 100 people off the street and run them through a **computerized axial tomography (CAT) scanner,** which can provide a very accurate picture of the adrenal gland, adrenal tumors will be found in 2% to 3% of people who otherwise feel totally fine. So before you do anything drastic, keep in mind that there's a background chance of finding something based on the statistics identified by medical studies.

What kind of tumor could your mother have had? There are several possibilities, and some are hereditary. But before we discuss this issue further, we should briefly review the architecture of the adrenal gland.

The adrenal gland is small, usually weighing less than an ounce or so. It has an outer layer called the **cortex,** and an inner layer called the **medulla.** A tumor can arise in either layer. When tumors arise in the outer layer, they tend to produce things that the outer layer normally makes anyway—for example, hormones such as cortisol (see Question 29) and aldosterone (a mineralocorticoid; see Question 91). These hormones, when made in abundance, can certainly raise your blood pressure. Tumors of the outer or cortical layer are usually sporadic (i.e., they just happen), and are not commonly hereditary.

When tumors arise in the inner layer of the adrenal gland, they normally make what the inner layer makes anyway—namely, adrenaline. These kinds of tumors, which are called pheochromocytomas (see Questions 16 and 21), do sometimes run in families.

Thus, if you know the kind of tumor your mother had, that information will help in answering this question. Otherwise, your doctor will assess your symptoms and perform some blood tests to determine whether you need a special radiology test to look

Computerized axial tomography (CAT) scanner

A machine that performs CAT type scans. CAT is an acronym that stands for Computerized Axial Tomogram or Tomography.

Cortex

Outermost layer. If you have ever shelled peas, the pod is the 'cortex' and the pea is the 'medulla' (see Medulla).

Medulla

(See Cortex). This is the inner portion of a gland.

for an adrenal tumor. Tumors in the outer layer of the adrenal gland tend to be associated with lower potassium values in the blood. Tumors in the inner layer tend to be more symptomatic—for example, they may be linked to sweating, heart racing, and pounding headaches. Tumors of the inner layer can also raise your blood sugar, occasionally to diabetic levels. As mentioned in Question 22, when a tumor is found in the inner layer of the adrenal gland, your doctor may recommend genetic testing given that these tumors do seem to have a family connection.

99. I see a psychiatrist for depression. Are there certain blood pressure medications or antidepressants I should be concerned about?

Many of the drugs used to treat depression work on centers of the brain that use chemicals such as adrenaline or its closely related cousins to communicate. As a result, there are some blood pressure side effects associated with **antidepressant** drugs. For example, some of these medications can cause your blood pressure to fall, especially when you change position.

Antidepressant

A medication used to treat depression.

Other antidepressants may cause your blood pressure to go up, because they work by blocking the enzymes that normally degrade adrenaline, which are called **monoamine oxidases (MAOs)**. When you're prescribed one of these MAO inhibitors, you will usually be given a list of foods to avoid so that you don't ingest tyramine (pronounced "tier-uh-meen"), a compound that can be a problem for your blood pressure because it acts in the adrenaline pathways in the body. Tyramine is found in Chianti wine, pickled herring, most cheeses, and pepperoni, for starters.

Monoamine oxidases

This term refers to enzymes which metabolize adrenaline. Low levels of adrenaline may be important in depression, and MAO drugs are given to increase the availability of adrenaline by blocking it's metabolism.

Here are some other specific drug interactions to watch for:

- Using antidepressants such as amitryptaline and alpha blockers: This combination has a tendency to produce big blood pressure reductions when you stand up (with some dizziness).

- Using antidepressants such as amitryptaline and diuretics and/or hydralazine: This combination can contribute to serious blood pressure reductions when standing up.
- Using lithium (e.g., Eskalith) and diuretics and/or ACE inhibitors: The blood pressure medications may increase the level of the lithium in the blood and produce toxicity.
- Using any antidepressant and clonidine: Clonidine can sometimes contribute to a depressed sensation, and it can interfere with drugs such as amitryptaline.
- Older beta blockers such as propranolol: These medications are thought to produce some depression because they are lipid soluble and hence accumulate in brain tissue, which is largely a lipid tissue.
- Reserpine: This older blood pressure medication has depression as a side effect when used in hypertension.
- MAO inhibitors: The usual recommendation is to avoid reserpine, clonidine, or methyldopa in conjunction with MAO inhibitors because they can precipitate a huge increase in blood pressure levels, called a hypertensive crisis.
- Selective serotonin reuptake inhibitors (SSRIs): These drugs, which include Zoloft and Paxil, don't usually cause problems with blood pressure.

100. There is so much information available about hypertension—where do I begin to learn more?

When I started to answer this question, just out of curiosity, I went to the Google website (www.google.com) and typed in "information about hypertension" (but I did not use the quotation marks). There were over 10 million "hits". Even the most determined hypertension student would be daunted by such a beginning.

In the next sections of this booklet I wrote a segment called " Literature and Other Sources of Information". In that section I and my nurse practitioner Virginia Ford (my gal Friday these past 14 years) have put together a series of books, websites, and useful articles that will help someone get more information on this important aspect of health. I am always interested in feedback, and you are welcome to send me an e-note at *townsend@mail.med.upenn.edu*. We have a fairly strict spam filter mechanism in place at the University of Pennsylvania, so be sure to put "100 Questions" in the subject line so I know to resurrect that message in case it ended up in the junk mailbox.

Who knows? Maybe there will be enough interest and new questions for a second edition or a spot on Oprah!

Thanks for reading!

Literature and Other Sources of Information

General Resources
Children Blood Pressure Levels by Age and Gender
You need Adobe Acrobat Reader for this one. The tables begin on page 10 of the
document itself,
Accessed May 11, 2007
http://www.nhlbi.nih.gov/health/prof/heart/hbp/hbp_ped.pdf

DASH Diet
Accessed May 7, 2007
http://dashdiet.org/dashdietbook.htm?google&gclid=CJWUraz6-
4sCFSMKGgodt2d7bg
There are loads of other sites on this topic, too. Google "DASH diet" and prepare
to upgrade your computer's memory to handle all the incoming information.

Hypertension in Children
Accessed May 31, 2007
www.nhlbi.nih.gov/guidelines/hypertension/child_tbl.htm

Hypertension in the Very Elderly
Accessed May 7, 2007
http://www.ncbi.nlm.nih.gov/entrez/query.fcgi?db=pubmed&cmd=Search&itool
=pubmed_AbstractPlus&term=%22Elliott+WJ%22%5BAuthor%5D
You might find it easier to access this document by typing http://www.pubmed.
com and then entering 15505119 in the open box (which is the Pub Med ID
number).

Joint National Committee 7th Report
This document is the biblical canon of hypertension care in the United States.
Accessed May 10, 2007
http://www.nhlbi.nih.gov/guidelines/hypertension/jnc7full.htm

Sleep Heart Health Study
Accessed May 7, 2007
http://www.jhucct.com/shhs/

Websites

Listed here are top picks from Yahoo and Google for hypertension patient information. User caveats: Some of the least credible websites are the more graphically attractive and enjoyable to "surf." Websites were rated from one heart to four hearts. The rating system is explained here:

♥♥♥♥ Four hearts indicates that (1) the information is researched, evidence-based, and appears unbiased; (2) the information is presented for the layperson in a simple format; (3) there are no advertisements; and (4) links are credible and relevant.

♥♥♥ Three hearts indicates that (1) the information is evidence-based, but may be biased (pharmaceutical sponsor); (2) the information is presented for the layperson and no input of personal information is required; (3) some advertisements are present but they are relevant to the information presented (i.e., a Pilates video); and (4) links are credible and relevant.

♥♥ Two hearts indicates that (1) most of the information is evidence-based, although appearing biased; (2) input of personal information is required; (3) information is presented for the layperson; and (4) advertisement links are relevant to the information provided, but some links are questionable.

♥ One heart indicates that (1) there is minimal credible information that is often critical of standard scientific medical treatment; (2) the information is difficult for layperson to process because of a plethora of advertisements; (3) the information does not include any evidence of efficacy and is potentially medically unsound; and (4) links are anecdotal in nature. Use at your own risk!

♥♥♥♥ www.patient.uptodate.com
Excellent evidence-based educational information, presented in an organized way, no advertising, and easy navigation to other reliable links.

♥♥♥♥ www.nhlbi.nih.com
Comprehensive evidence-based information with up-to-date research findings, links to Medline Plus to view a hypertension slideshow, a simple visual and sound hypertension lesson including basic physiology. No advertisements.

♥♥♥♥ www.hypertensionfoundation.org/
Offers a free download of Hypertension Patient Education pamphlets in Adobe Acrobat format or you can order booklets up to quantity of 25 by sending a self-addressed, stamped envelope with $1.00 postage.

♥ ♥ ♥ ♥ www.docguide.com
Hypertension information, medical news and alerts, discussion groups, related links, good presentation of target organs (click on brain, heart, vessels, eye, kidneys), short explanations, easy to navigate.

♥ ♥ ♥ ♥ www.patienteducationcenter.com
Sponsored by Medical Group Management Association. Its mission is to provide patients with multimedia access to reliable information at and beyond the point of care. Credible links, but does not include the American Society of Hypertension.

♥ ♥ ♥ http://my.webmd.com/
Credible information, some advertising for Glucerna and Reader's Digest recipes, information about Medicare Prescription benefits, sponsored by several pharmaceutical companies.

♥ ♥ ♥ www.americanheart.org/
Evidence-based information, hypertension news, risk calculator, heart-healthy tips, hypertension quiz, some relevant advertising (e.g., Omron, Coricidin HBP).

♥ ♥ ♥ www.intelihealth.com
Sponsored by an insurance company, features Harvard Medical School's Consumer Health Information, advertisements for a dental discount program. Provides comprehensive evidence-based information on herbal and alternative medications and treatments. Included is an interesting link on genetic testing.

♥ ♥ ♥ www.ash-us.org/
The American Society of Hypertension presents the most recent Joint National Committee guidelines (JNC 7). Comprehensive information on completed and ongoing hypertension trials, hypertension statistics, and antihypertensive drugs; requires a discerning reader.

♥ ♥ ♥ www.auburn.edu
Web page created by a Pharm.D. student. Gives evidence-based information in short bullet-format slides, but curiously the drug slide does not include diuretics. Gives a link to Lifeclinic for more information.

♥ ♥ ♥ www.CNN.com
Short bullet-format presentation on hypertension risk, symptoms, treatment, and prevention; advertisements for Pilates, pedometers, and thigh workout videos, among other products; links to a good site called Danger Zones that shows hy-

pertension's target organ disease points; also reports news items of the day. Fun to surf.

♥ ♥ www.lifeclinic.com
Credible information, need to sign up and give personal information but at no cost, includes advertisements (e.g., lose 10 pounds in four weeks), good section on hypertension tools, DASH diet, health tracking charts.

♥ ♥ www.bloodpressure.com
Links to Lifeclinic website; includes advertisements for a diet program, diabetes supplies, and medicines; section on "Hypertension Tools" (i.e., DASH diet), health charts, tracking logs; easy and fun to navigate; need to sign up and give some personal information but at no cost.

♥ ♥ www.heartcenteronline.com
Requires entering personal information, presents evidence-based information and education, sponsored by a pharmaceutical company.

♥ ♥ www.bioinstitute.com
Advertises unproven treatments, such as a special comb to massage pressure points on the head purported to lower blood pressure and special footpads to detoxify the body as you sleep, thereby lowering blood pressure.

♥ ♥ www.viableherbalsolutions.com
Advertises a plethora of herbal supplements called Pressure Ease: Natural High Blood Pressure Support.

♥ www.thesilentkillerexposed.com/
"Researcher accidentally stumbles upon all-natural secret to dropping your blood pressure through the door ... almost overnight ... guaranteed." Electronic manual for sale.

Newsletters

Tufts Health and Nutrition Letter
200 Boston Avenue, Suite 3500
Medford, MA 02144
Website: www.healthletter.tufts.edu

Mayo Clinic Health Letter
Subscription Services
P.O. Box 9302
Big Sandy, TX 75755-9302
Website: www.MayoClinic.com

The Medical Letter, Inc.
1000 Main Street
New Rochelle, NY 10801-7537
Website: www.medicalletter.org

Journal Watch Cardiology
Massachusetts Medical Society
800 Winter Street
Waltham, MA 02451-1413
Website: www.jwatch.org

Hypertension Health Information

American College of Cardiology
9111 Old Georgetown Road
Bethesda, MD 20814-1699
Telephone: (800) 253-4636, (301) 897-5400
Website: www.acc.org

American Heart Association
7272 Greenville Avenue
Dallas, TX 75231
Telephone: (800) 242-8721
Website: www.americanheart.org

American Society of Hypertension
148 Madison Ave, 5th Floor
New York, NY 10016
Telephone: (212) 696-9099
Website: www.ash-us.org

National Heart, Lung, and Blood Institute Information Center
P.O. Box 30105
Bethesda, MD 20824-0105

Telephone: (800) 575-WELL, (301) 592-8573
Website: www.nhlbi.nih.gov/health/infoctr/index/htm

Books

These books were listed as popular picks on Barnes and Noble and Amazon web searches for hypertension, hypertension education, and hypertension information. While most of these books present scientifically sound information, others favor the natural approach and seem more appropriate for pre-hypertensive and Stage 1 hypertensive patients; however, advice is not always targeted for this population. The information imparted may be misunderstood by hypertensive patients with more elevated blood pressures or by more fragile patients with comorbid conditions. Some of the titles might appear worrisome and undermine your confidence in your medical provider. Mixed messages are given—for example, work with your doctor, but don't take medicine. Prices may vary.

Rating Scale for Books

♥ ♥ ♥ ♥ Scientifically supported information
♥ ♥ ♥ Some scientifically supported information
♥ ♥ Minimal scientifically supported information
♥ No scientifically supported information

♥ ♥ ♥ ♥ Sheldon G. Sheps, M.D. *Mayo Clinic on High Blood Pressure* (2nd ed.). Rochester, MN: Mayo Clinic, 2003.
The author is a world-renowned hypertension specialist. This version is an updated edition with easy-to-understand information on the prevention and management of hypertension. Includes DASH diet and six-step fitness plan. Discusses the patient as an active partner with the provider. 208 pp. Hardcover $31.95/paperback $11.53.

♥ ♥ ♥ ♥ Thomas Moore and Mark Jenkins. *The DASH Diet for Hypertension*. New York: Pocket Books, 2003.
This diet was approved by the American Heart Association and the American Society of Hypertension. Two large clinical trials have shown that people who ate a DASH diet lost weight and had lower blood pressure, cholesterol, and insulin resistance readings. The diet is rich in fiber magnesium, potassium, calcium, and antioxidants, and low in refined sugar. It is easy to follow. 358 pp. Paperback $6.29.

♥ ♥ ♥ ♥ Alan L. Rubin, M.D. *High Blood Pressure for Dummies*. New York: For Dummies, 2002.

Information is nicely organized, and the book is fun and easy to read. Includes humorous cartoons. This book is endorsed by the American Society of Hypertension. 360 pp. Paperback $14.95.

♥♥♥♥ Mike Kirby, Neil Poulter, and Simon Thom. *Shared Care for Hypertension.* London: Isis Medical Media, 2001.
This book discusses major clinical aspects of hypertension and stresses the importance of joint participation between hospitals, providers, and patients in the delivery of care to patients with the chronic condition of hypertension. 270 pp. Paperback $49.95.

♥♥♥♥ Donald E. Hricik, Michael C. Smith, Wright Jackson, et al. *Hypertension Secrets.* Portland: Elsevier Science, 2001.
Contributors from Case Western Reserve University cover a broad range of information about hypertension. 153 pp. Paperback $36.95.

♥♥♥♥ William M. Manger and Ray W. Gifford. *100 Questions to Ask Your Doctor About Hypertension.* Malden, MA: Blackwell, 2000.
The authors and editors are leading authorities in hypertension and officers of the National Hypertension Association. The book introduces the fundamentals of high blood pressure and the latest treatments for a general audience. It encourages the reader to take an active role in his or her treatment, and provides a foundation for patient empowerment. 144 pp. Paperback $15.95.

♥♥♥ Julian Whitaker. *Reversing Hypertension: A Vital New Program to Prevent, Treat, and Reduce High Blood Pressure.* New York: Warner Books, 2001.
This book combines conventional and alternative therapies, and favors nondrug therapy—for example, diet, exercise, mineral supplements, water intake, and stress management. The author proposes his own plan to lower blood pressure and to avoid dependence on drugs. 336 pp. Hardcover $30.00/paperback $10.17.

♥♥♥ Mark C. Houston, Barry Fox, and Nadine Taylor. *What Your Doctor May Not Tell You About Hypertension: The Revolutionary Nutrition and Lifestyle Program to Help Fight High Blood Pressure.* New York: Warner Books, 2003.
This book uses very simple language, and outlines a healing program and 30-day food regimen offering nutritional and dietary aids. 384 pp. Paperback $10.17.

♥♥ Robert Rowan, M.D. *Control High Blood Pressure Without Drugs.* New York: Fireside, 2001.
Provides comprehensive information on achieving a healthier lifestyle and addresses current issues such as illegal drugs, alcohol, and impotence in hypertension. Gives

advice using natural remedies as safe and effective alternatives to prescription drugs, although also suggests working with the doctor. 368 pp. Paperback $10.50.

♥ ♥ Richard D. Moore, Ph.D. *The High Blood Pressure Solution* (2nd ed.). Portland: Inner Traditions, 2001.
The author discusses prevention of hypertension at the cellular level and advocates a special diet to keep potassium and sodium in proper balance. 400 pp. Paperback $16.95.

E-Book

♥♥♥♥ PM Medical Health News. *21st Century Complete Medical Guide to High Blood Pressure, Hypertension, Authoritative NIH and FDA Documents, Clinical References, and Practical Information for Patients and Physicians* (Two CD-ROM Superset). Progressive Management, March 2004. 76,332 pp. $29.99.

Other Teaching Tools

Pharmaceutical company representatives provide booklets, pamphlets, and visual aids to assist in hypertension education. Their phone numbers are listed in the *Physician's Desk Reference*.

Glossary

A

Acid reflux: when the sphincter which separates the stomach from the esophagus is lax, stomach acid leads backward, or 'refluxes' up the esophagus. This acid reflux causes heartburn and sometimes a narrowing or stricture in the esophagus that can interfere with swallowing.

Actuaries: tables of life insurance company data that typically evaluate factors involved in risks of dying. These factors include things like cigarette use, blood pressure and cholesterol levels.

Adrenal glands: the two small endocrine glands located just above the kidneys. The adrenal glands secrete sex hormones, cortisol, and adrenaline (epinephrine).

Adrenergic: related to adrenaline. The adrenergic portion of the involuntary nervous system is responsible for increasing heart rate and increasing blood pressure when stimulated.

Angina: a symptom of squeezing-type chest discomfort, often associated with physical exertion, that is associated with coronary artery blockage. The activity places extra demands on the heart and the blocked coronary circulation cannot supply the heart enough oxygen and nutrient to keep up which causes the 'ache' perceived as chest discomfort.

Angiotensinogen: a protein made by the liver and to a lesser extent the fat cells. This protein is ultimately metabolized by enzymes to yield angiotensin-II a very potent blood pressure raising hormone.

Anomolous Coronary Artery[1]: "the term coronary artery anomaly refers to a wide range of congenital abnormalities involving the origin, course, and structure of epicardial coronary arteries. By definition, these abnormalities occur in less than 1% of the general population. Coronary artery anomalies are frequently found in association with other major congenital cardiac defects."

Added by author: 'Epicardial' means on the surface of the heart. The problem is that there may be no evidence (like other heart problems such as leaky valves with murmurs) that a coronary artery arises from an unusual place. Sometimes the coronary arteries arise from the pulmonary artery, which means that the blood supplying the heart is already depleted of oxygen since the pulmonary arteries carry oxygen-poor blood to the lungs to replenish the oxygen supply. So, when additional oxygen need is required (for example by exercise), the 'cupboard is bare' creating a condition known as 'ischemia' or suffocation which can lead to heart attack or even sudden cardiac death.

---

1. With permission from: http://www.emedicine.com/MED/topic445.htm. Accessed May 5, 2007.

Antidepressant: a medication used to treat depression.

Arteriogram: a medical procedure in which dye is injected into a blood vessel. This is done to identify narrowing or to define an important aspect of anatomy such as presence of a tumor or a swelling (aneurysm) of the blood vessel.

Atherosclerosis & atherosclerotic: these terms refer to hardening of the artery usually from the build up of cholesterol plaque in the innermost lining of a vessel which can limit or block blood flow in that vessel.

B

Bariatric: pertaining to weight.

Biomarkers: a term applied to things we measure in the blood or urine that have relevance (good or bad) to disease. Some are hormones, some are proteins, and some are just small molecules that accumulate, or are depleted, in specific disease states. For example the good form of cholesterol, 'HDL-cholesterol', is a biomarker. See question 22 for others.

Biopsy: a piece of tissue removed from the body and examined for abnormalities.

Brainstem: the part of the brain that regulates dilation and constriction of blood vessels.

C

Cardiac output: the quantity of blood, usually expressed in liters/minute, pumped by the heart each minute.

Cardiovascular: relating to the heart or blood vessels.

CAT-scanner: a machine that performs CAT type scans. CAT is an acronym that stands for Computerized Axial To-

mogram or Tomography. The axial refers to the orientation of the X-Ray to the body (it is usually set to take an X-Ray that divides the body cross-sectionally instead of long-ways). The tomogram refers to sections. So a CAT scan basically takes a number of cross sectional X-Rays in sections that are each about 1/2 inch thick.

Cholesterol: a form of lipid important in heart disease. Cholesterol is the basis for sex hormones and bile, but it is also a substance that can accumulate in the lining of blood vessels and cause blockages.

Classes of blood pressure medications: there are about eight classes of blood pressure medicines (see Figure 2). ACE-inhibitors block the Angiotensin-Converting Enzyme which reduces the production of angiotensin-II. Angiotensin Receptor Blockers (ARBs) block the binding of angiotensin-II to its receptor (see Receptor) on the blood vessel cell. Alpha$_1$-blockers inhibit adrenaline effects on the blood vessel. Beta-blockers inhibit adrenaline effect on heart muscles. Alpha$_2$-agonists (like clonidine) suppress adrenergic activity. Calcium channel blockers directly relax arterial blood vessels by blocking channels through which calcium enters blood vessels cells. See 'Diuretics.' Vasodilators also directly relax blood vessels cells.

Clinical trials: this is considered the best way, or the "gold standard" to demonstrate the benefits of treatment. In a clinical trial a group of people with a finding (like hypertension) are randomly assigned one or another treatment (usually without the nature of the treatment being known to the doctors conducting the study or the patients taking the treatment: this is called "blinding") and followed for a long time to see if one treatment has better outcomes (like less strokes for example) compared with the other treatment.

Cortex: outermost layer. If you have ever shelled peas, the pod is the 'cortex' and the pea is the 'medulla' (see Medulla).

Cortisol: a hormone from the cortex of the adrenal gland which is produced to offset inflammation in the body.

D

Diastole or diastolic: the period of time when the heart is not actively contracting. In a blood pressure value like 134/76 mm Hg the "76" is the diastolic value (the 134 is the *systolic* value).

Diuretic: substance or medication that causes an increase in urine excretion. Caffeine is an example of a naturally occurring mild diuretic. Hydrochlorothiazide, or HCTZ, is an example of a prescription diuretic.

E

Echocardiogram: a sound wave test that provides a picture of the heart. It usually gives a measure of heart wall thickness, how well the valves work and how efficiently the heart contracts.

Electrocardiogram: a test of the electrical activity of the heart. Little sticky pads are placed at different places on the chest and the electrical activity of the heart is recorded on a piece of special paper. It is also known as an 'EKG' or an 'ECG'. It is used to diagnose things like heart attack and heart wall thickening.

Esophagus: the swallowing tube or passageway that connects the mouth with the stomach

F

Formulary: a listing of drugs or medications available for dispensing by either a pharmacy, a hospital or a prescription warehouse.

G

Gestational: having to do with pregnancy.

Glomerulus (singular)/**glomeruli** (plural): these are the tiny filter units in each kidney that initiate the formation of urine. In health they allow only the liquid part of blood to be filtered, and a barrier against protein or cells like red blood cells appearing in the urine.

H

HDL cholesterol: high-density lipoprotein cholesterol; also called the 'good' cholesterol. HDL cholesterol is thought to return cholesterol from places like blood vessel linings to the liver for excretion in the bile.

Hormones: chemicals made by glands like the adrenal glands or the pancreas that signal other tissue to function in a particular manner. For example insulin is a hormone made by the pancreas which, when released into the blood, stimulates the liver (and other tissues) to take up glucose (sugar) from the blood and store it. Hormones can also be made in the kidney.

Hypertension: also called high blood pressure. Hypertension is a circumstance in which a person's blood pressure has been shown to be consistently at or above 140/90 mm Hg. Hypertension is a leading risk factor for stroke, heart disease, kidney disease and peripheral circulation problems.

Hypertrophic Cardiomyopathy: cardiomyopathy is a condition in which the muscle of the heart is abnormal in the absence of an apparent cause. The normal alignment of muscle cells is absent and this abnormality is called **myocardial disarray.** *See Figure and full definition on page 155.

I

Inflammation & inflammatory: this term refers to the ability of a hormone, or a germ like a bacteria or virus, or some other influence to cause a reaction in the body that involves some aspect of the immune system. The result of this reaction is often a build up of scar or plaque. Inflammation is thought to play a big role in hardening of the arteries.

Insulin resistance: a situation in which insulin has difficulty promoting sugar uptake into body cells (the cells are resistant). High levels of insulin and sometimes blood sugar results. People with insulin resistance are higher risk for developing diabetes.

L

Lipids: generally considered these are the fats (or triglycerides) and cholesterol found in blood. Higher density lipids are the "good" fats and the lower density lipids are the "bad" fats.

Lipid profile: a blood test, usually done after fasting for 8 or more hours, that measures cholesterol (total, good and bad forms) and triglycerides levels.

M

Medulla: (see Cortex). This is the inner portion of a gland.

Mineralocorticoid: this term pertains to the salt, or mineral, retaining effects of adrenal cortical (see Cortex) hormones like aldosterone.

mm Hg: abbreviation for millimeters (mm) of mercury (chemical symbol is Hg), the units in which blood pressure is measured.

Mono-amine oxidases (MAOs): this term refers to enzymes which metabolize adrenaline. Low levels of adrenaline may be important in depression, and MAO drugs are given to increase the availability of adrenaline by blocking it's metabolism.

N

Nephropathy: pertaining to harmful effects on the kidney.

O

Occiput: the back part of the head or skull.

Optic: pertaining to the eye.

Osteoarthritis: inflammation and stiffness of the joints that usually occurs in older persons as a result of deterioration of the cartilage around the joints.

P

Pappiledema: swelling of the place in the eye where the nerves and blood supply of the retina enter the eye from the brain.

Parasympathetic: that part of the involuntary nervous system which balances the adrenaline or sympathetic effects.

When the parasympathetic nervous system is active heart rates are slower and blood pressure is lower.

Parenchymal: pertaining to the pulp or tissue of an organ. It usually refers to the entire organ or tissue, and is used to distinguish the organ from its blood vessel or 'vascular' side. For example we use renal parenchymal disease to say the problem **IS** the whole kidney, and renal vascular disease when the problem is the blood supply **TO** the kidney.

Placebo: usually an inactive substance that contains no medication or active ingredient to be given to participants in a clinical trial to determine the effectiveness of a particular medication or substance.

Plaque: an area of hardening in the blood vessel.

Preeclampsia: a situation, usually arising after the 20th week of pregnancy, characterized by increased blood pressure, ankle swelling, and proteinuria (see Proteinuria) in a pregnant woman.

Pre-hypertension: a term used when someone's blood pressure is consistently 120-139 mm Hg in the upper number (see Systolic) and/or 80-89 mm Hg in the lower number (see Diastolic).

Prescription: an instruction from a licensed clinician like a physician, an advanced practice nurse, a midwife, or a physician's assistant that provides for a medication or device to be issued by a pharmacy.

Prostaglandins: these are one of the many lipids in the body. They were originally isolated from the prostate gland (thus the name) but have since been found to be produced by many tissues. Some prostaglandins are helpful in that they reduce blood pressure and increase the excretion of salt in the urine. Other prostaglandins raise blood pressure, or cause platelets to stick together initiating a blood clot, or cause tissue inflammation as in the joint pain of Osteoarthritis (see Osteoarthritis).

Proteinuria: This term refers to the presence of protein in the urine. Protein is not usually detected in the urine of healthy individuals.

R

Receptor: this term usually refers to a protein that is anchored on the surface of a cell that specifically attracts a certain chemical or hormone. For example, the insulin receptor binds insulin from the blood stream and once the binding occurs, a series of reactions in the cell make possible the uptake of sugar (glucose) into that cell. The insulin receptor does not bind adrenaline, for example, so we typically say that receptors are choosy about who they are willing to partner with. Said another way we typically assert that receptors are specific in the ligands (chemicals/hormones) they bind.

Renal: pertaining to the kidney.

Resistance: a term carried over from the world of physics. In electricity there are three forces. There is a certain amount of moving force, a certain amount of flow, and certain amount of resistance to flow that are related by this formula: Force = Flow * Resistance. (The * is a math symbol for multiplication. Reading this aloud you would say "Force equals flow times resistance"). See Vascular Resistance.

Retinopathy: pertaining to harmful effects in the back of the eye (i.e. the retina).

S

Servo: a response system connected to other systems and dedicated to serving a purpose, like supporting blood pressure levels. Servos increase their activity when their target system is showing signs of insufficient activity. Servos dial back their influence when the system they serve shows signs of excessive activation.

Static: this term refers to something that is steady or unchanging

Sympathetic: this term refers to that part of the involuntary nervous system that increase heart rate and increases blood pressure.

Systole or systolic: the period when the heart is actively contracting. With a blood pressure like 126/88 mm Hg the 126 represents the systolic value (the 88 is the diastolic value).

T

Triglyceride: a type of fat, or lipid, that serves as the principal energy storage form of fat calories in the body. Triglycerides are stored in many tissues, but most notably in fat cells. Triglycerides circulate in the body in a particle called a Very Low Density Lipoprotein or VLDL. When VLDL particles are depleted of their triglycerides, they become Low Density Lipoproteins (LDL) which are very rich in the bad form of cholesterol.

V

Vascular: this term refers to blood vessels. It usually, but not always, refers to the artery type of blood vessels in particular.

Vascular resistance: this term refers to how hard it is to "push" the blood through the circulation. When resistance is high it takes more force to move blood through the tissues.

W

White Coat Hypertension: this term refers to someone whose blood pressure is high in a healthcare setting (like a doctor's office where it has been taken by someone in a "white coat") but it is lower at home or when evaluated by ambulatory blood pressure monitoring (See Question 11).

Hypertrophic Cardiomyopathy: *Reprinted with permission from Cardiomyopathy Association. Accessed May 5, 2007 from: http://www.cardiomyopathy. org/*

Cardiomyopathy is a condition in which the muscle of the heart is abnormal in the absence of an apparent cause. This terminology is purely descriptive and is based on the Latin derivation. There are four types of cardiomyopathy: Hypertrophic (HCM), Dilated (DCM), Restrictive (RCM) and Arrhythmogenic Right Ventricular (ARVC). The main feature of Hypertrophic Cardiomyopathy is an excessive thickening of the heart muscle (hypertrophy literally means to thicken). Heart muscle may thicken in normal individuals as a result of high blood pressure or prolonged athletic training. In Hypertrophic Cardiomyopathy,

however, the muscle thickening occurs without an obvious cause. In addition, microscopic examination of the heart muscle in Hypertrophic Cardiomyopathy shows that it is abnormal. The normal alignment of muscle cells is absent and this abnormality is called myocardial disarray (See Figure below).

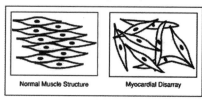

Normal Muscle Structure   Myocardial Disarray

Myocardial Disarray: these diagrams contrast the regular, parallel alignment of muscle cells in a normal heart (left)with the irregular, disorganised alignment of muscle cells or myocardial disarray (right) found in some parts of the heart in Hypertrophic Cardiomyopathy.

Index

page numbers followed by *f* denote figures; those followed by *t* denote tables

A

ABPM (ambulatory blood pressure monitor), 17–19, 47–48
ACE inhibitors. *See* Angiotensin-converting enzyme (ACE) inhibitors
Acetaminophen (Tylenol), increase in BP and, 85
Acid reflux, 81, 149
Actuaries, 149
Acupuncture, 60
Adrenal glands
    architecture of, 137
    defined, 22, 149
Adrenal tumors, 137–138
Adrenaline, 44, 46, 137
Adrenergic, 28, 149
African American patients
    damage to kidneys, 124
    effects of beta blocker medications, 84–85
    ethnic differences in BP response to medications, 86–87
    salt-sensitivity and, 87
Age, as predictor of hypertension, 8
Alcohol consumption
    effects on BP, 39, 62
    how much is safe to drink, 62–63, 62n
Aldomet (methyldopa), 133
Aldosterone, 137
Allergies, safe and unsafe medications, 123

Alpha-2 agonists, 53–54, 91*t*, 133
Alpha-blockers
    alpha-1 blockers, 74
    alpha-2 blockers, 74
    side effects, 91*t*, 138–139
Altace, 91*t*
Ambulatory blood pressure monitor (ABPM), 17–19, 47–48
American College of Cardiology, 145
American College of Physicians, 107
American Heart Association (AHA)
    contact information, 145
    high blood pressure research, 109
    when exercise is harmful, 55–56
American Society of Hypertension, 145
Amiloride, 45
Amitryptaline, and BP medications, 138–139
Amlodipine, 94
Anabolic steroid use, 50
AND-UA blood pressure kit, 15
Angina, 132, 149
Angiotensin-converting enzyme (ACE) inhibitors, 40–41, 74
    after heart attack, 128
    avoiding during pregnancy, 133
    combination therapy with a diuretic, 130–131
    ethnic differences in BP response to, 86–87
    to reduce effects of the renin system, 124–125
    side effects, 78, 91*t*
Angiotensin-receptor blockers (ABRs), 74, 78–79, 91*t*

after heart attack, 128

avoiding during pregnancy, 133

to reduce effects of the renin system, 124–125

Angiotensinogen, 40–41, 149

Angiotensinogen II and salt intake, 44

Ankle swelling, from medications, 91*t*, 93–95

Anomalous Coronary Artery, 56, 149, 149n

Anticancer agents, increase in BP and, 85

Antidepressant

BP side effects from, 138

defined, 15, 138

specific drug interactions, 138–139

Apressoline (hydralazine), 133

Arrythmogenic Right Ventricular Cardiomyopathy (ARVC), 152

Arteriogram, 113–115

consent form, signing, 115

defined, 150

procedure, 114

risks associated with, 114

Arthritis, exercising and, 55

Arthritis medications, increase in BP and, 85

Atenololl, 96

Atherosclerosis/atherosclerotic, 41, 150

Atkins Diet, 42

B

Bariatric, defined, 150

Bariatric surgery, 43

Baroreceptor system, 54, 115–116

Bench pressing, 50

Beta-blockers, 53–54, 74

after heart attack, 128

in pregnancy, 133

side effects, 91*t*

weight increase and, 93

Biomarkers

defined, 35, 150

inflammatory, from fat cells, 41

Biopsy, 136, 150

Birth defects, medication use in pregnancy and, 133–134

Blood evaluations, 112–113

Blood pressure, the basics. *See also* Hypertension, the basics

blood pressure machines in the super market, 19–20

blood pressure servos, 21–22, 23*f*, 109, 124–125

changes in during the day, 10–12

home readings

ambulatory blood pressure monitor (ABPM), 17–19

best home kit to use, 15–16, 17*f*

interpreting, 12

should you take them?, 13–14

ideal level, 68

importance of, 2

low BP, overtreatment and, 71–73

position of body when BP is taken, 31–32

relationship with the heart, 22

sitting quietly before taking, 11–12, 31

tests to predict development of hypertension, 34–35

at what age should children be checked, 30–31

what the numbers mean, 3–4

diastolic, 101

in older persons, 101–103

systolic, 101

when low BP becomes high BP, 8–9

wrist, taking blood pressure at, 116

Blood sugar monitoring, 112
Books about blood pressure, 146–148
Brain stem, 21, 150
Brand-name *vs.* generic drugs, 76–77
Breast feeding, medications during,
    134–135
Breathing machine that lowers BP,
    59–60

C
Calcium-channel blockers, side
    effects, 53–54, 91*t*
    effects of grapefruit juice and, 66
    in pregnancy, 133
    swollen ankles, 93–95
Capoten, 91*t*
Cardiac output, 44, 150
Cardiologist, consultation with,
    108–109
Cardiovascular
    defined, 35, 150
    risk factors, search for, 35
Cardizen (diltiazem), 91*t*, 94
Cardura, 91*t*
CAT-scanner, 137, 150
Catapres. *See* Clonidine (Catapres)
Children
    blood pressure values for, 6
    at what age should BP be
        checked, 30–31
Children Blood Pressure Levels by
    Age and Gender, 141
Chlorthalidone, erectal dysfunction
    and, 80
Cholesterol, 150
    defined, 9
    link with hypertension, 9–10
Classes of BP medications, 74, 150
Clinical trials, 31, 150–151
Clonidine (Catapres)
    with antidepressants, 139

dose-related effects, 70
    dry mouth, 70
Cocoa, lowering BP with, 98
Coffee drinking, 64–65
Computerized axial tomography
    (CAT) scanner, 137, 150
Constipation, from medications, 91*t*
Continuous positive airway pressure
    (CPAP), 58–59
Cortex, 137, 151, 152
Cortisol
    adrenal tumors and, 137
    defined, 46, 151
    function of, 46–47
Cough, from medications, 91, 91*t*
Cough-cold preparations, increase in
    BP and, 85
Coumadin (warfarin), 130
Cozaar, 91*t*
CPAP (continuous positive airway
    pressure), 58–59
Cyclosporine, 85
Cytochrome p-450-3A4 (CYP3A4),
    66

D
DASH diet, 42, 141
DCM (Dilated Cardiomyopathy),
    152
Dental work, controlling BP before,
    131–132
Diabetes and hypertension, 41
    drug-induced, 95–96
    goal of target organ preservation,
        122
    interaction with BP medications,
        83
    level of optimal BP treatment, 122
Diastole/diastolic, 101, 151
Dietary issues
    alcohol

effects on BP, 62
how much is safe to drink,
    62–63, 62n
coffee, 64–65
diet pills, effects on BP, 87–88
dietary supplements
    (neutraceuticals), 63–64
fish oil capsules, 65
grapefruit/grapefruit juice, 66
hypertension and, 7
salt intake (*See* Salt intake)
Dilated Cardiomyopathy (DCM),
    152
Diltiazem (Cardizen), 91*t*, 94
Diovan, 91*t*
Direct renin inhibitors (DRIs), 74
Diuretic, 91*t*
    defined, 45, 151
    in pregnancy, 133
Diuretic-induced diabetes, 95–96
Dizziness, from medications, 91*t*
Doxazosin, erectal dysfunction and,
    80
Dry mouth, 91*t*

E
E-book about blood pressure, 148
Echocardiogram, 117–118, 151
Elderly patients
    BP measurements, upper *vs.* lower
        numbers, 101–103
    effects of BP medications in,
        89–90
Electrocardiogram (EKG or ECG)
    defined, 60, 151
    frequency of, 113
    function of, 118–119
    signs of BP effects on the heart, 68
    tracings, 119, 119*f*
Endocrinologist, consultation with,
    109

Environmental link to hypertension, 7
Epicardial, 149
Esophagus, 81, 151
Exercise. *See also* Lifestyle changes
    with arthritis, 55
    can improve lipid metabolism, 39
    can reduce the chance of
        developing diabetes, 39
    effects on blood pressure
        medications, 22–23
    how it helps BP, 54–55
    jogging or running, 51
    perspiring, effect on BP, 51–52
    protects the target organs, 22
    reduction in BP and, 52
    safety of exercise with
        hypertension, 48–49
        knowing what is a safe level of,
            49–50
    stopping medication, 53–54
    walking, 57
    weight lifting, 50
    as a weight loss method, 43
    when exercise is harmful, 55–56
    when you should join a gym,
        56–57
Eyes, effects of hypertension on
    grade 1 retinopathy, 125–126
    grade 2 retinopathy, 126
    grade 3 retinopathy, 126
    grade 4 retinopathy (pappiledema),
        126
    the retina in hypertension, 127*f*

F
Fainting, while on medication, 72
Falling, while on medication, 72
Fat cells, 40–41
Fatigue, while on medication, 72–73,
    91*t*
Felodipine, 66, 94

Finger blood pressure kits, 16
Fish oil capsules, 65
Food and Drug Administration
    (FDA), 76–77
Foods, with high salt content, 45
Ford, Virginia, 140
Formulary, 100, 151

G
Ganglionic blockers, 74
Gastric banding, 43
Gastrointestinal (GI) bypass, 43
Gastrointestinal therapeutic system
    (GITS), 81–82
Generic drugs *vs.* brand-name, 76–77
Genetic link to hypertension, 7, 8
    testing for, 34–35
Gestation/gestational. *See also*
    Pregnancy
    defined, 24, 151
Glomerulus/glomeruli, 124, 151
Grapefruit-sensitive medications, 66

H
HCM (Hypertrophic
    Cardiomyopathy), 56, 152, 155
HCTZ (hydrochlorothiazide), 45,
    91*t*, 151
Headaches and hypertension, 33
Heart attack, BP medications and
    guidelines for hypertension care,
    127–128
    exceptions to, 128
    other medications, 128–129
Hemoglobin in the blood, testing for,
    113
High blood pressure. *See*
    Hypertension, the basics
High density lipoprotein (HDL)
    cholesterol, 39, 151
Hippel Lindau disease, 34

Home blood pressure readings
    ambulatory blood pressure
        monitor (ABPM), 17–19
    home kits, 15–16, 17*f*
    interpreting, 12
    should you take your own BP?,
        13–14
Hormones, 10, 40, 151
    adrenal, 137
    interaction of salt with, 44
House of God, The, 97
Hydralazine (Apressoline), 133
Hydrochlorothiazide (HCTZ), 45,
    91*t*, 151
Hydrodiural, 91*t*
Hypertension, the basics
    during and after pregnancy, 24–25
    causes of, 7–8
    curable, 25–27
    defined, 4, 151–152
    diagnosis of, 5
        being sure it is correct, 20–21
        number of readings for diagnosis,
            5–6
    pre-hypertension, 6
    threshold of values for, 4–5
    values for children, 6
    in the elderly, 101–103
    headaches and, 33–34
    high cholesterol and, 9–10
    medical history, discussing with
        your physician, 29–30
    only when under stress, 20–21
    primary, 22, 29
    processes that control BP, 21–23,
        23*f*
    secondary, 22, 29
    variability in readings, 27
    when low BP becomes high BP,
        8–9
    when sleeping, 27–28

where blood pressure medicines
work, 23*f*
white coat hypertension, 17–18,
20–21, 118, 154
Hypertension health information,
145–146
Hypertension in Children,
(document access), 141
Hypertension in the Very Elderly,
(document access), 141
Hypertension in the Very Elderly
Trial (HYVET), 89
Hypertensive crisis, 139
Hypertrophic Cardiomyopathy
(HCM), 56, 152, 155

I
Imitrex, 85
Inderal, side effects, 91*t*
Inflammation/inflammatory, 35, 41,
152
Information sources
books, 146–148
E-book, 148
general sources, 141
hypertension health information,
145–146
newsletters, 144–145
other teaching tools, 148
websites, 141–144
Insulin resistance, 54–55, 152
Involuntary nervous system, 27–28
Isopten (verapamil), 66, 91*t*, 94
Isradipine, 94

J
Jogging, safety of, 51
Johansen, "Jack Rabbit," 39
Joint National Committee, 52
Joint National Committee 7th
Report (document access), 141

Journal of Clinical Hypertension, 65
Journal Watch Cardiology, 145

K
Kidney(s)
biopsy of, 136
effects of hypertension on
ethnic differences, 124
kidney circulation, 124
markers of kidney damage,
testing for, 125
salt servo balance, 124–125
function, testing for, 112

L
Labetol (Normodyne, Trandate),
dose-related effects, 70
Lifestyle changes. *See also* Exercise
acupuncture, 60
limit alcohol consumption, 39
lose weight if overweight, 38
Resp-e-Rate device, 59–60
salt intake
how does my BP increase
interaction of with hormones
that raise BP, 44
through cardiac output, 44
how much salt is safe?, 44–45
reducing, 38
use of Morton's Lite Salt or sea
salt, 45–46
sleep apnea, 57–58
stress and hypertension, 46–47,
47*f*
weight loss and lower BP readings,
42–43
weight loss methods
alter your diet and exercise
patterns, 43
bariatric surgery, 44

medications that aid in weight
loss, 43–44
why additional weight causes BP
to go up, 40–41
Lightheadedness, while on
medications, 72
Lipid profile test, 49, 112, 152
Lipids, 10, 152
Lithium, and BP medications, 139
Loniten, 91*t*
Lying down while taking a pressure
reading, 31–32

M
Manual blood pressure cuff, 16, 17*f*
Mayo Clinic Health Letter, 145
Medical Letter, Inc., The, 145
Medications
adding a second medication,
83–84
advice from others, dealing with,
76
after a heart attack or heart failure
guidelines for hypertension care,
127–128
exceptions to, 128
other medications, 128–129
approval process, 97
beginning therapy, factors in the
decision, 68–69
classes of, 74
continued for life, 69
deciding which medications to
give, 103–104
diet pills, effects on BP, 87–88
discontinuing abruptly, effects of,
70–71
drug interactions with BP
medicines, 82–83
effects on sexual performance and
desire, 79–80

elderly patients, effects of BP
medications in, 89–90
formulary, 100
generic drugs *vs.* brand-name,
76–77
grapefruit juice, reactions with, 66
increased BP with
hypertensive medications, 84–85
other medications, 85
risk-benefit trade-off, 86
missing a dose, 70
news reports about, concerns
caused by, 96–98
overtreatment, signs of, 71–73
paying for, 77–78
alternative medication suggested
by insurer, 100–101
peak effect, 82
pharmacist list of adverse effects,
98–99
pregnancy and, 132–134
reduction in stroke incidence and,
130–131
shapes and sizes of, 81
side effects
angiotensin receptor blockers, 74
changing or discontinuing
because of, 75
deciding if the antihypertensive
medication is to blame, 92
direct renin inhibitors (DRIs), 74
drug-induced diabetes, 95–96
ganglionic blockers, 74
of major BP medications, 91*t*
opportunities for, 73
options if you need a certain
drug, 78–79
swollen ankles
associated with calcium-
channel blockers, 93–95
other cause of, 95

weight increase, 93
time of day for taking, 90–91
timed-release tablets, 81
trouble swallowing, remedies for,
    81–82
for weight loss, 43
where blood pressure medications
    work, 23*f*
withdrawing
    if you exercise regularly, 53–54
    issues to consider, 69–70
Medulla, 137, 152
Methyldopa (Aldomet), 133
Milk/plasma (M/P) ratio, 134–135
Mineral balance, monitoring,
    112–113
Mineralocorticoid, 128, 152
Mineralocorticoid antagonists
    (MRAs), 128
mm Hg, 4–5, 152
Monoamine oxidases (MAOs)
    antidepressants and, 139
    defined, 152
    effect on BP, 138
Morton's Lite Salt, 45–46
Myocardial disarray, 155, 155*f*

N

National Heart, Lung, and Blood
    Institute of the NIH, 109,
    127–128
Information Center, 145–146
Nature/nurture connection to
    hypertension, 8
Nephrologist, consultation with,
    108–109
Nephropathy, 64, 152
Nervous system, involuntary, 27–28
Neurofibromatosis, 34
Neutraceuticals, 64
Newsletters, 144–145

Nicadipine, 94
Nifedipine, 66, 94
Nifedipine-GITS (Procardia GITS),
    81
Nisoldipine, 66, 94
Norvasc, 91*t*

O

Occiput, 33, 153
Omron blood pressure kit, 15
Optic, 126, 153
Organ transplant drugs, increase in
    BP and, 85
Osteoarthritis, 111, 153
Overweight, hypertension and, 7

P

Pappiledema, 126, 153
Parasympathetic, 28, 153
Parenchymal kidney disease, 26, 153
Paxil, 139
Paying for medications, 77–78
    alternative medication suggested
        by insurer, 100–101
Peak effect, medications, 82
Peridopril Protection Against
    Recurrent Stroke Study
    (PROGRESS), 131
Perspiring while exercising, effect on
    BP, 51–52
Phenotype, 34
Pheochromocytoma, 25–26, 34, 137
Physician/provider issues
    complaints, how the doctor
        handles them, 110–111
    different doctors, different
        medications, 106–107
    echocardiogram, 117–118
    Rheos system, 115–116
    taking BP readings at the wrist,
        116

testing for hypertension
arteriogram, 113–115
blood tests, 112–113
electrocardiogram, 112, 118–119, 119*f*
urine tests, 113
type of specialist to consult, 108–109
when the medication doesn't help, 109–110
when to consult a hypertension specialist, 107–108
PIER (Physicians Information and Education Resource), 108
Placebo, 78, 153
Plaque, 10, 153
Polysomnogram (PSG), 58
Position of body when BP is taken, 31–32
Potassium intake, 45–46
Potassium levels, low, from medications, 91*t*
Pre-hypertension, 6, 153
Preeclampsia, 24, 153
Pregnancy
antihypertensive medications in case-controlled studies, 132
safe/unsafe, 132
hypertension that may become permanent, 24–25
types of hypertension associated with, 24
Prescription, 66, 153
Procardia, 91*t*
Procardia GITS (nifedipine-GITS), 81
PROGRESS (Peridopril Protection Against Recurrent Stroke Study), 131
Propranolol, 139
Prostaglandin, 65, 66

Proteinuria
defined, 135, 153
significance of, 135–136
testing blood and urine, 136

R

RCM (Restricted Cardiomyopathy), 152
Receptor, 153–154
Redux, 87–88
Renal, 113, 154
Renal vascular disease, 113–114
Renin system, 124–125
Reserpine, 139
Resistance, 3, 154
Resources for hypertension patients. *See* Information sources
Resp-e-Rate device, 59–60
Restricted Cardiomyopathy (RCM), 152
Retinopathy
defined, 154
grade 1, 125–126
grade 2, 126
grade 3, 126
grade 4 (pappiledema), 126
the retina in hypertension, 127*f*
Rheos system, 115–116
Rimonabant, 43
Running, safety of, 51

S

S-T and T wave changes, EKG, 119, 119*f*
Salt intake
African American patients and, 87
angiotensinogen II and, 44
dietary issues, 22, 23*f*
foods with high salt content, 45
how much salt is safe?, 44–45

use of Morton's Lite Salt or sea
salt, 45–46
how does my BP increase
interaction of with hormones
that raise BP, 44
through cardiac output, 44
reducing, 38
salt servo balance, 124–125
Sea salt, use of, 45–46
Selective serotonin reuptake
inhibitors (SSRIs), 139
Servos, 21–22, 23*f*, 109, 154
Sexual performance and desire,
effects of medications on, 79–80
Shem, Samuel, 97
SHEP (Systolic Hypertension in the
Elderly Program), 101–102
Sitting while taking a pressure
reading, 11–12, 30–31
Sleep apnea and hypertension, 57–58
Sleep Heart Health Study, 58, 141
South Beach Diet, 42
Spironolactone, 45
SSRIs (selective serotonin reuptake
inhibitors), 139
Static, 11, 154
Statins, effect of grapefruit on, 66
Stress and hypertension, 20–21,
46–47, 47*f*
Stroke
incidence of, 130
reduction in stroke incidence, BP
medications and, 130–131
Super market blood pressure
machines, 19–20
Supplements, dietary, 64
Surgery, taking your medications
before, 129–130
Swallowing, trouble with, remedies
for, 81–82
Swelling of ankles, from medications,
91*t*, 93–95

Sympathetic, 28, 154
Systole/systolic, 101, 154
Systolic Hypertension in the Elderly
Program (SHEP), 101–102

T
Tacrolimus, 85
Thalidomide, 134
Time of day for taking medications,
90–91
Timed-release tablets, 81
Treatment of Mild Hypertension
Study (TOMHS), 80
Triamterene, 45
Triglyceride, 10, 11, 154
Tufts Health and Nutrition Letter,
144
Tumors of the adrenal gland, 137–
138
Tylenol (acetaminophen), increase in
BP and, 85
Tyramine, 138

U
Upper arm blood pressure kits, 15–16
Urine testing, 112

V
Vascular, 56, 154
Vascular resistance, 102, 154
Vasodilators, 74, 91*t*
Verapamil (Isopten), 66, 91*t*, 94
Vioxx, 83
Virginia
the ABPM pressure monitor and
stress, 47–48
acceptance of her problem, 27
diagnosis of hypertension, 9
lifestyle changes, 39–40
primary care doctor, 107
resting before taking BP, 12
taking home readings, 14–15

weight-loss pills, 88–89

Visual analog stress scale, 47f

W

Walking, 57

Warfarin (Coumadin), 130

Websites, patient information, 141–144

Weight gain, from medications, 93

Weight lifting, 50

Weight/weight loss

    effect of diet pills on BP, 87–88

    exercise, as a weight loss method, 43

    lose weight if overweight, 38

    weight-cycling, 88

    weight loss and lower BP readings, 42–43

    weight loss methods

        alter your diet and exercise patterns, 43

        bariatric surgery, 44

        medications that aid in weight loss, 43–44, 87–88

        why additional weight causes BP to go up, 40–41

White coat hypertension, 17–18, 20–21, 118, 154

Withdrawal of medications

    if you exercise regularly, 53–54

    issues to consider, 69–70

Wrist, taking blood pressure at, 116

X

Xenical, 88

Z

Zoloft, 139